健康照护师职业培训系列教材
总策划　何振喜
总主编　王社芬

英语日常口语对话

刘丹丹　主　编

中国科学技术出版社
·北　京·

图书在版编目（CIP）数据

英语日常口语对话／刘丹丹主编．—北京：中国科学技术出版社，2022.12
健康照护师职业培训系列教材
ISBN 978 - 7 - 5046 - 9374 - 7

Ⅰ.①英…　Ⅱ.①刘…　Ⅲ.①英语 - 口语 - 职业培训 - 教材　Ⅳ.①R319.9

中国版本图书馆 CIP 数据核字（2021）第 249220 号

本书编委会

主　编　刘丹丹

副主编　罗　萍　邱孝丰

编　委（按姓氏笔划排序）

马慧娟　王贺佳　邓珺文　李　静

李慧颖　赵　婧　强　薇

主要人物介绍

　　本书以健康照护师王素琴（英文名 Susan Wang）在李先生家工作为背景，围绕王素琴和李先生一家的日常生活，以对话为形式，介绍了健康照护师所需的日常英语知识。全书内容包括饮食、生活起居、室内游戏、户外活动及生病和健康照护五个部分。

健康照护师 Susan Wang 王素琴	姐姐 Ann Li 李安安	弟弟 Philip Li 李飞飞	妈妈 Mrs. Li 李太太
爸爸 Mr. Li 李先生	姥姥 Mrs. Zhao 赵太太	姥爷 Mr. Zhao 赵先生	健康照护师 Tracy 崔蕾

绘图　周佳仪

目 录

CHAPTER FIVE　HEALTH CARE

CHAPTER ONE   HAVE A MEAL

FEEL THIRSTY

对话

Mom：Are you thirsty?
妈妈：你口渴吗？

Ann：Yes，very much！
安安：是的，非常渴！

Mom：You may drink some water.
妈妈：你可以喝些水。

Ann：OK. I'd like a glass of water now. But Mom，why don't I feel thirsty after drinking water?
安安：好的，我要喝一杯水。妈妈，为什么喝水就不渴了呢？

Mom：Because you need water to replenish your body.
妈妈：因为喝水可以补充身体的水分。

Ann：What else can replenish the body?
安安：还有什么可以补充身体的水分呢？

Mom：Juice，milk and so on.
妈妈：果汁、牛奶等都可以的。

Ann：I see.
安安：我记住了。

词汇

thirsty [ˈθɜːsti] adj. 口渴的
replenish [rɪˈplenɪʃ] vt. 补充

EAT FRUIT

对话

Ann：What fruit is it?
安安：这是什么水果？

Dad：This is a banana. You can peel it and eat it.
爸爸：这是香蕉，把皮剥开就可以吃。

Ann：What other fruits must be peeled before eating?
安安：还有什么水果需要剥皮吃？

Dad：Oranges and grapes.
爸爸：橙子和葡萄。

Ann：What fruits can be eaten without peeling?
安安：有什么水果是可以带着皮吃的呢？

Dad：Let me see，for example，apples，peaches and pears，but you need to wash them before eating.
爸爸：让我想一想，比如苹果、桃和梨。不过，这些水果要清洗干净再吃哦。

1

词汇

peel [piːl] vt. 剥皮
skin [skɪn] n. 外皮

WASH THE APPLE

对话

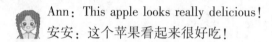 Ann：This apple looks really delicious！
安安：这个苹果看起来很好吃！

Mom：Yes, the apple is red and big. It looks delicious！
妈妈：是的，这个苹果又红又大，看起来很美味！

Ann：Mom, this apple is too big for me to eat.
安安：妈妈，这个苹果太大了，我吃不完。

Mom：How about cutting it in half so that we can share them？
妈妈：我把这个苹果切成两半，我们一起分享好吗？

Ann：That is a great idea！
安安：这可真是个好主意！

Mom：Don't forget to wash the apple before you eat it！
妈妈：吃苹果之前要记得清洗哦！

Ann：Let's wash the apple together.
安安：我们来一起清洗苹果吧。

词汇

delicious [dɪˈlɪʃəs] adj. 美味的
share [ʃeə(r)] v. 分享

MAKE FRUIT TRAY

对话

 Ann：I'd like to bring some fruits to the New Year Party.
安安：新年派对我想给大家带些水果。

 Mom：How about making a fruit tray？
妈妈：做个果盘怎么样？

 Ann：Great！ But I'm not sure how to make it. What do I need？
安安：好棒！但是我不会做，需要些什么呢？

 Mom：You'll need a pretty platter and at least three different fruits.
妈妈：你需要一个漂亮的大浅盘和至少三种不同水果。

 Ann：So easy！ Let's make a fruit tray！
安安：这么简单！让我们来做个果盘吧！

 Mom：Chop the melon and slice the kiwi fruit.
妈妈：甜瓜切块，猕猴桃切片。

 Ann：How about the strawberries？
安安：草莓呢？

 Mom：Don't slice the strawberries if you want them to look fresh and delicious. Leave them whole to preserve their freshness.
妈妈：你如果想要草莓看起来更新鲜、美味，就不要把它们切开。完整的草莓才能保持新鲜。

词汇

tray ［treɪ］ n. 盘子

platter ［ˈplætə(r)］ n. 大浅盘

chop ［tʃɒp］ v. 切

freshness ［freʃnəs］ n. 新鲜

EAT DINNER

对话

Grandma：Dinner is ready!

姥姥：晚饭好啦!

Ann：Wow, what a delicious meal!

安安：哇,好丰盛的饭菜!

Grandma：I made dishes with meat and vegetables.

姥姥：我做了肉和素菜。

Ann：And toast. It's great!

安安：还有烤面包,真棒!

Mom：This is beef stew with potatoes. It's very delicious. Have a taste.

妈妈：这是土豆炖牛肉,很美味,你尝尝。

Ann：Is this a new dish to have potatoes with beef?

安安：土豆和牛肉搭配,这是新的菜式吗?

Mom：No, it's a traditional Chinese dish. There are many dishes that match vegetables with meat like this! Such as radish with lamb, celery with pork, and tofu with fish. These are all good matches.

妈妈：不是的,这是中国的传统美

食。像这样把蔬菜和肉搭配的菜还有很多呢!比如萝卜和羊肉、芹菜和猪肉、豆腐和鱼肉,这些都是不错的搭配。

词汇

taste ［teɪst］ n. (用来品尝的)一点儿,少量

stew ［stjuː］ n. 炖煮的菜肴

celery ［ˈseləri］ n. 芹菜

match ［mætʃ］ n. 搭配

USE TABLEWARE

对话

Ann：What do you use to eat soup?

安安：你用什么餐具喝汤?

Mom：I use a spoon for soup.

妈妈：喝汤要用勺子。

Ann：What do you use to eat steaks?

安安：用什么吃牛排呢?

Mom：I need a knife and a fork for steaks.

妈妈：吃牛排要用刀和叉。

Ann：What do you use to eat dumplings?

安安：用什么吃饺子呢?

Mom：Dumplings are traditional Chinese dish. Chinese people are accustomed to eating with chopsticks.

妈妈：饺子是中国的传统美食。中国人习惯用筷子吃饭。

Ann：Which hand should I use for chopsticks?

安安：我应该用哪只手拿筷子？

Mom：We usually use our right hand.
妈妈：通常用右手。

Ann：What about the knife and fork?
安安：那刀和叉呢？

Mom：Usually left hand for fork and right hand for knife, you see, like this.
妈妈：通常是左手叉、右手刀，你看，像这样。

词汇

chopstick［'tʃɒpstɪk］n. 筷子
steak［steɪk］n. 牛排

HAVE A BALANCED DIET

对话

Ann：I'm hungry. What do we have today? I'd like to eat a lot of meat.
安安：好饿，今天我们吃什么呢？我想吃很多很多的肉。

Grandpa：That's not a good idea. Eating much more meat than vegetables will cause nutritional deficiency and constipation!
姥爷：那可不行哦，肉多菜少会引起营养缺乏和便秘哦！

Ann：I should eat both meat and vegetables!
安安：我应该吃肉也吃菜！

Grandpa：That's right. A balanced diet is very important.
姥爷：这就对了，膳食平衡非常

重要。

Ann：I want to be a good girl who is not picky.
安安：我要做一个不挑食的好宝宝。

Grandpa：Yes, vegetables with meat are nutritious and healthy!
姥爷：对，吃菜配肉，营养又健康！

词汇

nutritional［nju'trɪʃənl］adj. 营养的
deficiency［dɪ'fɪʃnsi］n. 缺乏
constipation［ˌkɒnstɪ'peɪʃn］n. 便秘
balanced［'bælənst］adj. 平衡的
diet［'daɪət］n. 饮食
picky［'pɪki］adj. 挑食的

KEEP A BLAND DIET

对话

Susan：Are you enjoying your meal?
素琴：饭菜合胃口吗？

Dad：It looks very good, but it tastes a little salty!
爸爸：卖相非常好，就是吃起来有点咸！

Susan：I'll put less salt next time.
素琴：我下次少放点盐。

Dad：Eating less salt is good for our health.
爸爸：少吃盐对身体好。

Susan：Yes. Taking too much salt may lead to high blood pressure.
素琴：是的。吃多了盐可能会导致血压升高。

Dad：We should take less sugar too.
爸爸：糖也要少吃。

Susan：Taking too much sugar will cause diabetes.
素琴：糖吃多了容易患糖尿病。

词汇

salty ［ˈsɔːlti］ adj. 咸的
diabetes ［ˌdaɪəˈbiːtiːz］ n. 糖尿病
high blood pressure 高血压
taste ［teɪst］ vt. 尝

REFILL YOUR BOWL

对话

Susan：Have you had enough to eat?
素琴：你吃饱了吗?

Ann：I haven't had enough.
安安：我还没吃饱。

Susan：Eat more!
素琴：多吃点哦!

Ann：May I have some more rice?
安安：可以再来些米饭吗?

Susan：Here you are. Do you want to eat more vegetables?
素琴：给你。再吃点菜吗?

Ann：No, thanks, I haven't finished mine yet.
安安：不用了，我的菜还没吃完呢。

Susan：Do you want to mix rice and chicken?
素琴：把米饭和鸡肉掺在一起好吗?

Ann：No, please put the chicken in another bowl.
安安：不要，请把鸡肉放在另一个碗里。

Susan：Sure, honey.
素琴：好的，宝贝。

词汇

refill ［ˌriːˈfɪl］ v. 重新装满
bowl ［bəʊl］ n. 碗

KEEP A MODERATE DIET

对话

Mom：It's a good habit to eat properly.
妈妈：适量饮食是好习惯。

Ann：Why?
安安：为什么?

Susan：Because eating too much is not only easy to gain weight, but also easy to get sick.
素琴：因为吃得太多容易长胖，而且容易得病哦。

Mom：You will spoil your appetite if you eat a lot.
妈妈：吃太多会破坏你的食欲。

Ann：What will happen if eating less?
安安：吃少了会怎么样?

Susan：It may cause malnutrition and hinder your body growth.
素琴：会营养不良，会影响身体成长。

Ann：I get it.
安安：我知道了。

词汇

habit［ˈhæbɪt］n. 习惯
properly［ˈprɒpəli］adv. 适量地
malnutrition［ˌmælnjuːˈtrɪʃn］n. 营养不良

SIT DOWN TO EAT

对话

Susan：Ann, take a seat while you're eating.
素琴：安安，吃饭的时候要坐下来。

Ann：But I want to watch cartoons.
安安：可是我想看动画片。

Susan：Do not distract yourself while eating.
素琴：吃饭的时候不要分心。

Ann：Can I eat in bed?
安安：我可以在床上吃饭吗？

Susan：Lying and eating in bed can cause choking easily.
素琴：躺在床上吃饭容易噎到，不安全。

Ann：Can I eat while playing games?
安安：我可以边做游戏边吃饭吗？

Susan：It's easy to get indigestion. Sit by the table and eat quietly, so that your stomach feels comfortable.
素琴：这样容易消化不良。吃饭就要安静地坐在餐桌旁，这样胃才会舒服。

Ann：I won't run around, I will sit down by the table and eat well.
安安：我不乱跑了，我会坐在餐桌旁，好好吃饭。

词汇

cartoon［kɑːˈtuːn］n. 动画片
indigestion［ˌɪndɪˈdʒestʃən］n. 消化不良
comfortable［ˈkʌmftəbl］adj. 舒服的
run around　东奔西跑

USE NAPKINS

对话

Philip：Please hand me a napkin. There are some oil stains on my hands.
飞飞：请给我一张餐巾纸。我的手上有些油渍。

Dad：Here you are. You'd better wash your hands.
爸爸：给你。你最好把手洗一下。

Philip：It's not enough. Can I have another one?
飞飞：不够，我可以再来一张吗？

Dad：Here you are.
爸爸：给你。

Philip：Thank you Dad. It is still not enough. I need more napkins.
飞飞：谢谢爸爸。还不够用。我需要更多的餐巾纸。

Dad：After using one side of the napkin, you can fold it and use the other side.
爸爸：餐巾纸用完一面，可以折叠一下，再用另一面。

Philip：How do you fold it? Can you show me?
飞飞：怎么折叠？你能做一下吗？

Dad：Let me show you.
爸爸：我来教你。

Philip：Now I know how to make full use of a napkin.
飞飞：现在我会用餐巾纸了。

词汇

napkin［'næpkɪn］n. 餐巾纸
stain［steɪn］n. 污渍
fold［fəʊld］v. 折叠

DON'T WATCH TV WHILE EATING

对话

Mom：Ann, it's time for dinner.
妈妈：安安，吃饭了。

Ann：I don't want to eat anything.
安安：我不想吃。

Mom：Why don't you want to eat?
妈妈：为什么不想吃饭？

Ann：Because I want to watch cartoons.
安安：因为我想看动画片。

Mom：How about watching TV after dinner?
妈妈：吃完饭再看电视怎么样？

Ann：I want to watch TV now!
安安：我现在就想看电视！

Mom：I made your favorite dish, Sweet and Sour Chicken.
妈妈：我做了你最喜欢吃的菜，糖醋鸡。

Ann：I'd like to eat right now!
安安：我现在要吃饭！

词汇

sweet［swiːt］adj. 甜的
sour［'saʊə(r)］adj. 酸的

EAT BY YOURSELF

对话

Philip：Grandma, feed me please!
飞飞：姥姥，喂我吃！

Grandma：A good kid always does things on his own and eats by himself. You are a good kid, aren't you?
姥姥：好孩子自己的事自己做，饭也要自己吃哦。你是个好孩子，对吗？

Philip：I am, and I will eat by myself. I will also tell the kids in my kindergarten to eat by themselves.
飞飞：我是个好孩子，我要自己吃饭。我还要告诉我幼儿园的小朋友们，要自己吃饭。

Grandma：You are such a good boy.
姥姥：你真是个好孩子。

Philip：Does my teacher like me to eat by myself?
飞飞：老师会喜欢我自己吃饭吗？

Grandma：Yes, she does.
姥姥：她会的。

词汇

feed［fiːd］v. 喂养
kid［kɪd］n. 小孩

kindergarten ［ˈkɪndəɡɑːtn］ n. 幼儿园

CLEANING UP

对话

 Susan：Mrs. Zhao, have you had enough to eat?
素琴：赵女士，您吃饱了吗？

 Grandma：Yes, I have done very well! Let's clean the table and wash the dishes.
姥姥：是的，吃饱了！我们收拾桌子和洗碗吧。

 Susan：OK. Let me put the plates in the kitchen sink.
素琴：好的。我来把盘子放到厨房水槽里。

 Grandma：Hold the plates gently and steadily.
姥姥：盘子要轻轻拿稳。

 Susan：Next, clean up the table.
素琴：接着清理桌子。

 Grandma：Let me help you hold the trash can.
姥姥：我帮你拿着垃圾桶。

 Grandma：Then, set up the chairs.
素琴：还要把椅子摆放整齐。

 Grandma：Thank you.
姥姥：谢谢。

词汇

hold ［həʊld］ vt. 拿着
steadily ［ˈstedəli］ adv. 平稳地

DIET DURING ILLNESS

对话

 Grandma：I had a fever today.
姥姥：我今天发烧了。

 Susan：You need to drink more water, eat light food and hot soup. You will recover soon.
素琴：你需要多喝水、吃清淡的食物、喝热汤。这样很快就会好的。

 Grandma：I don't want to eat or drink anything. I have a bitter taste in my mouth.
姥姥：我什么都吃不下，也喝不下，我的嘴巴里是苦的。

 Susan：Let me make you some watermelon juice.
素琴：我给您做个西瓜汁吧。

 Grandma：Thank you. I'd like a glass of watermelon juice.
姥姥：谢谢你。我想喝杯西瓜汁。

 Susan：I'm going to make it right now.
素琴：我现在就给您做。

 Grandma：Thanks.
姥姥：谢谢。

词汇

have a fever 发烧
light food 清淡饮食
bitter ［ˈbɪtə(r)］ adj. 苦的
taste ［teɪst］ n. 味道

CHECK THE BEST–BEFORE DATE

对话

Dad：The bread tastes a little bit sour.
爸爸：这个面包吃着有点酸味。

Susan：Let me have a look.
素琴：让我看看。

Dad：Here you are.
爸爸：给你。

Susan：Don't eat it! It's gone way past its best-before date. You'd better check the expiry date before eating.
素琴：别吃了！早过期了。吃东西之前要查看保质期。

Dad：How long is the best-before date of the bread?
爸爸：这个面包的保质期是几天？

Susan：In summer, it is 3 days.
素琴：夏天的话，保质期是3天。

Dad：Oh, it's too short.
爸爸：哦，这么短。

Susan：While in winter, it is 7 days.
素琴：冬天的话，是7天。

Dad：Shall we store bread in the fridge? So the best-before date will be 7 days.
爸爸：那我们是不是可以把面包放在冰箱里储存？这样保质期就是7天了。

Susan：OK.
素琴：好的。

词汇

best-before date　保存限期
fridge ［frɪdʒ］ n. 电冰箱
store ［stɔː(r)］ v. 储存

STORAGE FOOD

对话

Susan：Do you want some yogurt?
素琴：你想喝酸奶吗？

Philip：Where is the yogurt?
飞飞：哪里有酸奶？

Susan：In the fridge. The yogurt must be refrigerated or it will go bad quickly.
素琴：在冰箱里。酸奶需要冷藏，否则很容易变质。

Philip：The fridge is really useful in summer. Can we store all the food in the fridge?
飞飞：在夏天冰箱真有用。所有的食物都可以放在冰箱里吗？

Susan：No, you shouldn't. Some fruits cannot be kept in the fridge, such as bananas and mangoes.
素琴：不可以，有些水果就不能放在冰箱里，比如香蕉和芒果。

Philip：Can we store papayas in the fridge?
飞飞：木瓜可以放在冰箱里吗？

Mom：Papayas cannot be stored in the fridge too.
妈妈：木瓜也不能放在冰箱里储存。

Philip：There is a papaya in the fridge. I'll get it out.

飞飞：冰箱里有一个木瓜，我把它拿出来。

Susan：We can make a yogurt papaya salad.

素琴：我们做一个酸奶木瓜沙拉。

Philip：That's a great idea.

飞飞：好主意。

词汇

mango ['mæŋgəʊ] n. 芒果

papaya [pə'paɪə] n. 木瓜

WASH YOUR HANDS

对话

Susan：Wash your hands before meals.
素琴：饭前要洗手哦。

Ann：Why?
安安：为什么呢？

Susan：It's easy to have loose bowls after eating food with dirty hands.
素琴：用不卫生的双手吃了食物容易腹泻。

Ann：All right. I'm going to wash my hands.
安安：好，我现在就去洗手。

Susan：Do you know that you must wash your hands after eating?
素琴：你知道吃完饭也要洗手吗？

Ann：Yes I know. I need to wash my greasy hands after eating.

安安：我知道的。吃完饭需要洗洗油手。

Susan：You are right.
素琴：安安说得对。

Ann：From now on, I will wash my hands before and after eating a meal.
安安：以后我吃饭前和吃饭后都要洗手。

Susan：Then you will develop a good habit!
素琴：这样你就养成了一个好习惯！

词汇

loose bowels　腹泻

develop a habit　养成一个习惯

TAKE A WALK

对话

Susan：Mr. Zhao, You can't do strenuous exercise after meals!
素琴：赵先生，刚吃完饭不能剧烈运动的！

Grandpa：What is considered strenuous exercise?
姥爷：什么样的运动是剧烈运动呢？

Susan：Such as running and playing basketball.
素琴：比如跑步和打篮球。

Grandpa：Can we go for a walk after supper?
姥爷：那吃完晚饭可以散步吗？

Susan：Of course, walking after supper is good for digestion.

素琴：当然，晚饭后散步有利于消化。

Grandpa：I'm going to take a walk. It's so comfortable to go for a walk after supper.
姥爷：我要去散步了。吃完晚饭散步好舒服。

Susan：Yes, it is.
素琴：是的。

Grandpa：My friend and I used to play basketball right after lunch. No wonder I got a stomachache.
姥爷：我和朋友们过去经常吃完午饭就打篮球。难怪我会胃疼。

词汇

strenuous ['strenjuəs] adj. 剧烈的
stomachache ['stʌməkeɪk] n. 胃痛

BROKE A PLATE

对话

Grandma：I broke a plate by accident today.
姥姥：我今天不小心打碎了一个盘子。

Susan：Did you hurt yourself?
素琴：您伤到自己没有？

Grandma：No, I didn't. I swept the pieces together and dumped them in the garbage bin.
姥姥：没有，我把碎片扫到了一起，倒进垃圾桶里了。

Susan：Allow me to inspect the floor to see if there are any missing pieces.
素琴：我来检查一下，看看有没有遗漏的碎片在地板上。

Grandma：It is necessary for you to take a look. Oh my poor eyesight, I am worried that I did not clean it thoroughly.
姥姥：很有必要看一看。我视力不好，正担心清理不彻底呢。

Susan：Don't worry, leave it to me. I will also warn the children not to walk on the floor with bare feet.
素琴：别担心，交给我吧。我也会告诉孩子们，不要光着脚在地板上走。

词汇

sweep [swiːp] v. 扫去
eyesight ['aɪsaɪt] n. 视力
bare [beə(r)] adj. 赤裸的

BAKE POTATOES

对话

Dad：I have bought some potatoes. How do we cook them?
爸爸：土豆买回来了，我们怎么做呢？

Susan：How about stir-fried shredded potatoes?
素琴：炒土豆丝怎样？

Grandpa：I'd like stir-fried shredded potatoes.
姥爷：我想吃炒土豆丝。

Susan：No problem, I can make both baked potatoes and stir-fried shredded potatoes.

素琴：没问题，我可以做烤土豆和炒土豆丝两种。

Grandpa：You shouldn't trouble yourself to make two dishes with potatoes.

姥爷：你不用这么麻烦，把土豆做成两种菜。

Susan：No trouble at all.

素琴：一点儿不麻烦。

Grandpa：Thank you, Susan.

姥爷：谢谢素琴。

词汇

fried [fraɪd] adj. 油炸的
bake [beɪk] v. 烘焙

HAVE DINNER

对话

Grandpa：It's already seven o'clock!

姥爷：已经七点了！

Grandma：Yes, it's too late.

姥姥：是呀，都这么晚了。

Grandpa：Shall we have dinner now?

姥爷：我们现在吃晚饭可以吗？

Susan：Dinner is ready.

素琴：晚餐准备好了。

Grandpa：Why didn't Ann come back yet?

姥爷：安安怎么还没回来？

Grandma：I forgot to tell you that she's having a party tonight and will not be back for dinner.

姥姥：我忘记告诉你，她今晚有派对，不回来吃晚饭了。

Grandpa：Is there anything for Ann to eat when she comes back at night?

姥爷：安安晚上回来有吃的吗？

Susan：There are dumplings in the fridge. I will make dumplings for her if she is hungry.

素琴：冰箱里有饺子。如果她饿了，我给她煮饺子吃。

Grandpa：All right.

姥爷：好的。

词汇

already [ɔːlˈredi] adv. 已经
hungry [ˈhʌŋgri] adj. 饥饿的

CHAPTER TWO   DAILY ACTIVITIES

PUT ON SHOES

对话

Ann：Mom，can we go out to play?
安安：妈妈，我们能出去玩吗？

Philip：Mom，I'd love to play on the swing.
飞飞：妈妈，我喜欢玩荡秋千。

Mom：Of course，but we must change our shoes before we go outside.
妈妈：当然可以了，但是出门前，我们需要换鞋。

Susan：Do you need some help?
素琴：需要帮忙吗？

Philip：No，thanks. I can do it. Is it right?
飞飞：不，谢谢。我可以的。这样穿对吗？

Susan：Phil，well done. You can put on shoes by yourself.
素琴：飞飞，做得不错。你能自己穿鞋子了。

词汇

swing［swɪŋ］n. 秋千

TAKE OFF SHOES

对话

Ann：It's so much fun that I don't want to go home.
安安：真的是太好玩了，我都不想回家了。

Philip：Me neither. I really enjoy swinging. Mom，can we play outside tomorrow?
飞飞：我也不想回家了。我真的是太喜欢荡秋千了。妈妈，我们明天还能出来玩吗？

Mom：Sure. It's getting late today. Let's go home.
妈妈：当然可以，今天已经很晚了。我们回家吧。

Ann：Susan，could you help me take off my shoes? I can't untie my shoelaces.
安安：素琴，你能帮我脱鞋子吗？我解不开鞋带了。

Susan：OK，no problem. Just untie them in this direction.
素琴：好的，没问题。只要顺着这个方向解开就可以了。

Ann：Susan，thank you.
安安：素琴，谢谢你。

Susan：You're welcome.
素琴：不客气。

词汇

untie [ʌnˈtaɪ] vt. 解开
shoelace [ˈʃuːleɪs] n. 鞋带

词汇

shot [ʃɒt] n. 尝试
doll [dɒl] n. 洋娃娃
smog [smɒg] n. 烟雾
wear [weə(r)] vt. 穿；戴

WEAR A MASK

对话

Philip：Dad, shall we go shopping today?
飞飞：爸爸，今天我们能出去逛街吗？

Ann：Dad, I want a Peppa doll.
安安：爸爸，我想要一个佩奇布娃娃。

Dad：OK, but there is smog today. We must wear anti-smog face masks before going outside.
爸爸：可以，不过今天有雾霾，出门前我们必须戴好防雾霾口罩。

Ann：Susan, can you help us?
安安：素琴，你能帮我们一下吗？

Susan：I'd love to. Let me show you how to wear a mask properly, and you'll be able to give it a shot, OK?
素琴：我非常愿意。我给你们示范一下佩戴口罩的正确方法，然后你们试一下，好吗？

Ann：Wow! Susan, I can wear a mask by myself!
安安：哇！素琴，我可以自己戴口罩啦！

Susan：Well done!
素琴：做得真棒！

WEAR GLOVES

对话

Ann：Susan, the snow is heavy. Can we go out to play?
安安：素琴，外面的雪好大啊，我们能出去玩吗？

Philip：I'd like to make snowmen.
飞飞：我想堆雪人。

Susan：Okay, let's ask Mom.
素琴：好的，那我们问问妈妈吧。

Ann：Mom, could we go outside to play?
安安：妈妈，我们能去外面玩吗？

Philip：Mom, I'd like to make snowmen.
飞飞：妈妈，我想去堆雪人。

Mom：Okay, let's make snowmen and have a snowball fight. It's very cold outside, so we have to wear hats and gloves before going outside.
妈妈：好的，我们去堆雪人，打雪仗吧。外面天气很冷，所以出门前我们需要先戴帽子和手套。

Ann：We're going to play in the snow!
安安：我们要去玩雪啦！

词汇

snowman ['snəʊmæn] n. 雪人（复数形式为 snowmen）

snowball ['snəʊbɔːl] n. 雪球

glove [glʌv] n. 手套

TIDY UP THE ROOM

对话

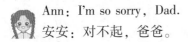

Dad：Honey, your room is a mess. There are toys everywhere.

爸爸：宝贝，你的房间真的是太乱了，玩具到处都是。

Ann：I'm so sorry, Dad.

安安：对不起，爸爸。

Dad：It's OK. Let's tidy up the room. Susan and I will give you a hand.

爸爸：没关系，我们整理一下房间吧。我和素琴都会帮你。

Susan：Let's do it together.

素琴：让我们一起整理吧。

Ann：Thanks Dad. Thanks Susan.

安安：谢谢爸爸，谢谢素琴。

Ann：I'm going to sort out the toys and put them in the box.

安安：我来整理玩具并把它们收到箱子里。

Philip：I'm going to make the bed.

飞飞：我来整理床铺。

词汇

mess [mes] n. 杂乱

GET VACCINATED

对话

Mom：Ann, you should get vaccinated today.

妈妈：安安，今天你得去打疫苗了。

Ann：Mom, I don't want to go. It hurts. I'm very scared.

安安：妈妈，我不想去。会疼的。我很害怕。

Mom：It's all right, honey. It does hurt a little during the shot, but I will be there for you all the time, OK?

妈妈：没事的，宝贝。打针时是有一点疼，但妈妈会一直陪着你，好吗？

Ann：Does Susan go with us?

安安：素琴和我们一起去吗？

Mom：Of course. Susan and I will be there for you.

妈妈：当然，妈妈和素琴都会陪着你。

Susan：We can play a counting game when you get the shot. You can count from 1 to 5. When you count 5, the vaccine has been done. And you will find that it doesn't hurt that much.

素琴：当你打疫苗的时候，我们可以玩个数数的游戏。你可以从1数到5。当你数到5时，疫苗就打完了。你会发现打疫苗并没有想象中那么疼。

Mom：Honey, let's go!

妈妈：宝贝，我们出发吧！

15

词汇

vaccinate ['væksɪneɪt] v. 给······注射疫苗

scared [skeəd] adj. 害怕的

shot [ʃɒt] n. 注射

count [kaʊnt] v. 数数

WAIT YOUR TURN

对话

Ann：Susan, I'm very hungry. Can we go to the nearest McDonald's to buy hamburgers and fried chips?
安安：素琴，我好饿。我们能去最近的麦当劳买汉堡和薯条吗?

Susan：Sure. There are a lot of people in the McDonald's and we'll have to wait in line.
素琴：可以，麦当劳人很多，我们要排队。

Ann：Can we cut in line?
安安：我们能插队吗?

Susan：Waiting in line to order food is a virtue. So we should wait.
素琴：排队点餐是一种美德，所以我们要排队等候。

Ann：I've got it.
安安：我明白了。

Susan：The ordering speed of McDonald's is very fast, and you'll have delicious hamburgers and fried chips soon.
素琴：麦当劳的点餐速度很快，一会儿你就能吃到好吃的汉堡和薯条啦。

词汇

hamburger ['hæmbɜːɡə(r)] n. 汉堡包

virtue ['vɜːtʃuː] n. 美德

CROSS THE STREET

对话

Philip：Mom, the green light will not turn to red until 10 seconds later. Let's run.
飞飞：妈妈，绿灯 10 秒钟后就会变成红灯，我们快跑吧。

Mom：Phil, the time is not enough. It's too dangerous if we run a red light. Let's wait for the next green light.
妈妈：飞飞，时间不够，如果我们闯了红灯就太危险了。我们还是等下一次绿灯吧。

Philip：OK, Mom. Let's wait on the sidewalk.
飞飞：好的，妈妈，我们去人行道等吧。

Mom：Phil, when we cross the street, could you walk on my right side and hold my hand tightly? Don't run away, OK?
妈妈：飞飞，过马路时，你站在我的右手边，紧紧握着我的手，不要乱跑，好吗?

Philip：OK, I promise.
飞飞：好的，我答应你。

Mom：You've learned how to cross the street properly and safely.

妈妈：你已经学会如何正确、安全地过马路啦。

词汇

sidewalk ［'saɪdwɔːk］n. 人行道
tightly ［'taɪtli］adv. 紧紧地
properly ［'prɒpəli］adv. 正确地

SAY SORRY

对话

 Philip：Susan, I'm sorry. I broke my mother's favorite vase by accident when I was playing football.
飞飞：素琴，对不起。我踢足球时不小心把妈妈最喜欢的花瓶打碎了。

 Susan：It's OK. I'm sure Mom won't blame you. Did the broken pieces hurt you?
素琴：没关系。我相信妈妈不会责怪你的。碎片伤到你了吗？

Philip：No, I was not hurt.
飞飞：没有，我没受伤。

Susan：Thank goodness, you did not hurt yourself. First things first, I'll sort out the broken vase, and you'll go and apologize to Mom, OK?
素琴：谢天谢地，你没有受伤。当务之急，我先收拾一下破碎的花瓶。你去向妈妈道歉，好吗？

Philip：OK, Susan. Thank you for your help.
飞飞：好的，素琴。谢谢你的帮忙。

 Philip：Mom, I'm so sorry. I just broke your favorite vase by accident.
飞飞：妈妈，对不起。我刚刚不小心把你最喜欢的花瓶打碎了。

 Mom：It doesn't matter. I can buy a new vase. Fortunately, you didn't hurt yourself.
妈妈：没关系。我可以买一个新的花瓶。幸好你没有受伤。

词汇

vase ［vɑːz］n. 花瓶
first things first 当务之急
apologize ［ə'pɒlədʒaɪz］vi. 道歉

HAVE A TASTE

对话

Ann：This strawberry cake looks so delicious!
安安：这个草莓味蛋糕看起来不错呀！

Philip：This is the birthday cake for Dad, so we can't eat it now.
飞飞：这是给爸爸的生日蛋糕，我们现在不能吃。

Ann：I know, but I really want to eat it.
安安：我知道，但是我真的好想吃啊。

 Susan：Ann, let's ask Mom if it is OK to have a taste.
素琴：安安，我们去问问妈妈能不能尝一口。

Ann：Mom, Could I eat the cake now? I'd like to have a bite of it.

安安：妈妈，我现在可以吃蛋糕吗？我想吃一口。

Mom：I think you can have a bite. I'm sure Dad won't mind.

妈妈：你可以吃一口。我相信爸爸不会介意。

Ann：Hooray!

安安：好棒！

Susan：I'm going to cut a small slice of the cake. Have a taste of it.

素琴：我切一小块蛋糕。你尝一尝。

Ann：Thank you. Wow, it's so delicious.

安安：谢谢。哇，太好吃了。

词汇

birthday [ˈbɜːθdeɪ] n. 生日

SHARE A SECRET

对话

Ann：Susan, tomorrow is my mother's birthday. I have prepared a birthday present for her. It's a secret. Can you promise me that you won't tell anyone until tomorrow?

安安：素琴，明天是我妈妈的生日，我为她准备了生日礼物。这是个秘密，你能保证明天之前不能告诉任何人吗？

Susan：Yes, I promise. It's our little secret. Can I have a look?

素琴：好的，我保证。这是我们的小秘密。我能看一下吗？

Ann：I drew a family picture of Dad, Mom, Phil, you and me.

安安：我画了一幅全家福，有爸爸、妈妈、飞飞、你和我。

Susan：Wow, Ann, you're really good at drawing.

素琴：哇，安安，你真的很擅长画画。

Ann：Thank you!

安安：谢谢！

Susan：The pretty girl with the pigtail is Ann, am I right?

素琴：这个扎着辫子的漂亮女孩是安安，对吗？

Ann：Yes, yes!

安安：对呀，对呀！

Susan：The cute boy in the suit is Phil, isn't he?

素琴：这个穿着西装的可爱男孩是飞飞，是吗？

Ann：Yes, it's Phil.

安安：是的，是飞飞。

Susan：I think this is me.

素琴：我想，这是我吧。

Ann：Yes, Susan, it's you.

安安：对，素琴，是你。

Susan：Ann, thank you. I'm so happy to be in your family picture.

素琴：安安，谢谢你，能出现在你的全家福里我真的特别开心。

Ann：Susan, you will always be my best friend.

安安：素琴，你永远是我最好的朋友。

词汇

secret ［ˈsiːkrət］ n. 秘密
draw ［drɔː］ v. 画
pigtail ［ˈpɪgteɪl］ n. 辫子

RECONCILE DISPUTES

对话

Ann：Phil，this is the Barbie doll Mom bought for me. Is she beautiful?
安安：飞飞，这是妈妈送给我的芭比娃娃，好看吗?

Philip：No, it isn't. My Super Flying that Dad gave me is better.
飞飞：不好看。爸爸送给我的超级飞侠更好。

Ann：The Barbie is better.
安安：芭比娃娃更好。

Philip：The Super Flying is better.
飞飞：超级飞侠更好。

Ann：Let's go ask Susan which toy is better.
安安：我们去问问素琴，哪个玩具更好。

Susan：Let me have a look. Well, the Barbie has miraculous dress-changing magic. The Super Flying is a mailman who helps to make dreams come true. They have unique characteristics, so I think the Barbie and the Super Flying are equally great.
素琴：让我看一看。嗯，芭比娃娃拥

有神奇的换装魔法。超级飞侠是帮助实现梦想的邮递员。他们各有各的特点，所以我觉得芭比娃娃和超级飞侠都很棒。

Ann：Yes, I like Phil's Super Flying as well.
安安：对呀，我也喜欢飞飞的超级飞侠。

Philip：I think Ann's Barbie doll is very beautiful.
飞飞：我觉得安安的芭比娃娃很漂亮。

Ann：Thanks, Phil. Let's share our toys and play together.
安安：谢谢飞飞。我们分享玩具，一起玩吧。

词汇

dispute ［dɪˈspjuːt］ n. 争吵
reconcile ［ˈrekənsaɪl］ v. 使和解
miraculous ［mɪˈrækjələs］ adj. 神奇的
mailman ［ˈmeɪlmæn］ n. 邮递员
characteristic ［kærəktəˈrɪstɪk］ n. 特点
dream ［driːm］ n. 梦想

TO BURP

对话

Philip：Ann, you drink juice too fast. You might burp. See, you're burping. Haha!
飞飞：安安，你果汁喝得太快了，可能会打嗝。看吧，你打嗝了，哈哈!

Susan：Phil, don't laugh at Ann. You should drink juice slowly as well.

Otherwise you might burp too.

素琴：飞飞，不要嘲笑安安，你也要慢一点喝果汁。否则，你可能也会打嗝。

Philip：I won't burp. Hic…Hic…
飞飞：我不会打嗝的。嗝……嗝……

Ann：Haha! Phil is burping, too.
安安：哈哈！飞飞也打嗝了。

Susan：All of us should drink juice slowly next time.
素琴：下次我们都要慢一点喝果汁。

词汇

burp ［bɜːp］ v. 打嗝
otherwise ［ˈʌðəwaɪz］ adv. 否则

GO OUT IN THE RAIN

对话

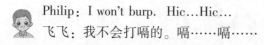

Philip：I don't have any pencils or erasers. Can we go out and buy some?
飞飞：我的铅笔和橡皮没有了。我们能出去买点吗？

Susan：OK. Let's ask Mom.
素琴：好的，我们问问妈妈吧。

Philip：Mom, we want to buy some pencils and erasers, could we?
飞飞：妈妈，我们想去买铅笔和橡皮，可以吗？

Mom：Yes, of course. But now it's raining outside. Don't catch a cold.
妈妈：好的，当然可以。不过现在外面下着雨，别感冒。

Philip：Okay, Mom.
飞飞：好的，妈妈。

Susan：Phil, let's put on our raincoats and boots, and get umbrellas, OK?
素琴：飞飞，我们穿上雨衣和雨靴，拿上雨伞，好吗？

Philip：Okay, Susan. Thank you.
飞飞：好的，素琴，谢谢你。

词汇

raincoat ［ˈreɪnkəʊt］ n. 雨衣
boot ［buːt］ n. 靴子
umbrella ［ʌmˈbrelə］ n. 雨伞

MEET GUESTS

对话

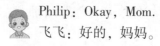

Dad：Ann, Phil, this is my colleague, John. John, this is my daughter Ann, and this is my son Phil.
爸爸：安安，飞飞，这是我的同事约翰。约翰，这是我的女儿安安，这是我的儿子飞飞。

Ann：Hello, Uncle John.
安安：你好，约翰叔叔。

Philip：Hello, Uncle John.
飞飞：你好，约翰叔叔。

John：Hello, Ann. Hello, Phil. Nice to meet you. These are the gifts for you.
约翰：你好安安。你好飞飞。很高兴认识你们。这是送给你们的礼物。

Ann：Thank you, Uncle John.
安安：谢谢你，约翰叔叔。

Philip：Thank you, Uncle John.
飞飞：谢谢你，约翰叔叔。

John：You're welcome.
约翰：不客气。

Dad：Ann, Phil, could you play with toys in your room? John and I have a lot of work to talk about.
爸爸：安安，飞飞，你们能去房间里玩玩具吗？我和约翰叔叔还有很多工作要谈。

Ann：Okay, Dad.
安安：好的，爸爸。

词汇

colleague ['kɒliːg] n. 同事

MEASURING CHILDREN'S HEIGHT AND WEIGHT

对话

Mom：Ann, we need to go to the community hospital for a routine physical examination. We will have your height and weight measured, OK?
妈妈：安安，我们需要去社区医院做常规体检，需要测量身高和体重，好吗？

Ann：Mom, does it hurt?
安安：妈妈，会疼吗？

Mom：Don't worry, Ann. It doesn't hurt at all.
妈妈：不用担心，安安，一点也不疼。

Susan：Ann, when your height and weight are taken, you just need to step on the scale and hold still for 3 seconds, OK?
素琴：安安，给你测量身高和体重时，你只需要站在秤上，保持不动，等3秒钟，好吗？

Ann：I see. Thank you, Susan. Mom, let's go and have a body check up now!
安安：我知道了。谢谢你，素琴。妈妈，我们现在去体检吧！

Mom：Okay, Ann. I will be with you.
妈妈：好的，安安．我会陪在你身边的。

Ann：Thank you, Mom.
安安：谢谢你，妈妈。

词汇

community [kə'mjuːnəti] n. 社区
routine [ruː'tiːn] adj. 常规的
physical ['fɪzɪkl] adj. 身体的
examination [ɪgˌzæmɪ'neɪʃn] n. 检查

BUY CLOTHES

对话

Mom：Phil, you've grown much taller lately. The shirt is too small to cover your belly.
妈妈：飞飞，你最近又长高了许多。这件衬衫太小了，都露肚子了。

Philip：Mom, but I really like this shirt.

飞飞：妈妈，我真的很喜欢这件衬衫。

Mom：We can go to the mall to see if there is a similar one.

妈妈：我们可以去商场看看有没有同款。

Philip：That's great, Mom. Will Susan go with us?

飞飞：太好了，妈妈。素琴和我们一起去吗？

Mom：Yes, She will.

妈妈：是的，她和我们一起去。

Susan：Phil, I will look around to see if there is a similar one and you could try on other shirts.

素琴：飞飞，我会去找同样的衬衫，你可以试试其他的衬衫。

Philip：OK. Let's go!

飞飞：好的。我们出发吧！

词汇

belly［'beli］n. 腹部
mall［mɔːl］n. 商场

DO HANDICRAFT

对话

Philip：Susan, today my homework is to make a paper castle. But I'm not sure how to make it.

飞飞：素琴，我今天的作业是做一个纸的城堡。但是我不知道怎么做。

Susan：Phil, don't worry. Let's ask Mom for help, she is good at it.

素琴：飞飞，别担心。我们请妈妈帮忙吧，她很擅长做这个。

Philip：That's fantastic.

飞飞：那太好了。

Susan：Let's go find Mom now!

素琴：我们现在去找妈妈吧！

Philip：Mom, I need to build a paper castle. Could you help us?

飞飞：妈妈，我需要建一座纸城堡。你可以帮助我们吗？

Mom：No problem. Before building the castle, we need some materials, such as cartons, colored pens and golden powder.

妈妈：没问题。在盖城堡之前，我们需要些材料，如硬纸盒、彩笔和金粉。

Philip：OK, we'll get the materials ready right away.

飞飞：好的，我们会马上准备好材料的。

Susan：I know where to find those materials. Let's look for them right now.

素琴：我知道哪里可以找到这些材料。现在我们去找吧。

Philip：Thank you, Susan.

飞飞：谢谢你，素琴。

词汇

handicraft［'hændikrɑːft］n. 手工
castle［'kɑːsl］n. 城堡
carton［'kɑːtn］n. 硬纸盒
material［mə'tɪəriəl］n. 材料

MAKE A CALL

对话

Ann：Susan, I miss grandma very much. I haven't seen her for a long time.

安安：素琴，我非常想念姥姥，我已经好久没有见到她了。

Susan：Yes, we haven't seen her for almost two months, since the last family dinner on Mid-Autumn Day.

素琴：是的，自从上次中秋节家宴，差不多有2个月没有见过她。

Ann：I miss her. I miss her chocolate cake.

安安：我好想念她，想念她做的巧克力蛋糕。

Susan：Ann, although we can't see her right now, you can call her.

素琴：安安，虽然我们现在不能马上见到她，但是你可以给她打电话啊。

Ann：Yes, you're right. I'm going to call grandma. Do you know her phone number?

安安：是的，你说得对。我要给姥姥打电话。你知道她的电话号码吗?

Susan：It's 1806655112.

素琴：电话号码是 1806655112。

Ann：Hello, is this grandma?

安安：你好，是姥姥吗?

Grandma：This is Grandma speaking. Honey, I miss you so much.

姥姥：我是姥姥。宝贝，我非常想你.

词汇

chocolate [ˈtʃɒklət] n. 巧克力

BE UNHAPPY

对话

Philip：Susan, come on. Why doesn't my goldfish move?

飞飞：素琴，你快来呀。我的金鱼为什么不动了呢?

Susan：Don't worry, Phil. Let me have a look. I'm sorry to say that the goldfish seems to be sick.

素琴：别着急，飞飞。让我看看。很抱歉，金鱼好像生病了。

Philip：Why does my goldfish get sick? Susan, what can I do to help the goldfish?

飞飞：我的金鱼为什么会生病呢？素琴，我要怎么做才能帮助金鱼呢?

Susan：Don't be so sad, Phil. I don't think it's a big problem.

素琴：别太伤心，飞飞。我觉得不是什么大问题。

Mom：Phil, my honey, why do you look unhappy today?

妈妈：飞飞，我的宝贝，你今天怎么看起来不开心呢?

Philip：Mom, my goldfish seems to be sick. I'm very worried.

飞飞：妈妈，我的金鱼好像生病了。我很担心。

Mom：Oh, poor goldfish. Phil, don't worry. We can take it to see the vet uncle Yang.

妈妈：噢，可怜的金鱼。飞飞，别着急。我们可以带它去找宠物医生杨叔叔。

Philip：Let's go right away.

飞飞：我们马上出发吧。

词汇

unhappy [ʌnˈhæpi] adj. 不快乐的
goldfish [ˈgəʊldfɪʃ] n. 金鱼
vet [vet] n. 兽医

SHARE TOYS

对话

Ann：Phil, your racing model is really cool. Could I play with it?

安安：飞飞，你的赛车模型真的是太帅了，我可以玩一下吗？

Philip：No, you will break it.

飞飞：不可以，你会把它弄坏的。

Ann：Phil, I don't like you. I wouldn't play with you anymore.

安安：飞飞，我不喜欢你了。我再也不和你玩了。

Susan：Ann, what's the matter?

素琴：安安，怎么啦？

Ann：Phil doesn't want me to play with his racing car.

安安：飞飞不想让我玩儿他的赛车。

Susan：You should share toys with each other. I promise that I will protect the car with Ann. We wouldn't break it. Could you please share your toy with Ann?

素琴：你们要互相分享玩具。我保证会和安安一起保护好赛车。不会弄坏它。你能和安安分享一下你的玩具吗？

Philip：All right. Ann, you can play it now. Don't break it.

飞飞：好吧。安安，你可以玩了。别弄坏了。

Ann：OK, Phil. I promise.

安安：好的，飞飞。我保证。

词汇

racing [ˈreɪsɪŋ] adj. 速度比赛
model [ˈmɒdl] n. 模型

GET UP

对话

Mom：Rise and shine, still dreaming children? It's time to get up.

妈妈：天亮啦，孩子们还在做梦吗？该起床啦。

Philip：Ten more minutes, Mom.

飞飞：我想再睡十分钟，妈妈。

Mom：It's already 8 o'clock. Wake up, or you will be late for kindergarten.

妈妈：已经八点了。起床啦，否则去幼儿园就迟到啦。

Ann：You don't need to wake me up. I'm already up.

安安：你不用叫我起床，我已经起来了。

Dad：Did you sleep well?

爸爸：你昨晚睡得好吗？

Philip：I'm still sleepy.

飞飞：我还是好困。

Ann：I had a good dream. Mom, do you want to hear about my dream?

安安：我做了个好梦。妈妈，你想听吗？

Mom：Sure.

妈妈：好呀。

词汇

dream ［driːm］v. 做梦
minute ［ˈmɪnɪt］n. 分钟
sleepy ［ˈsliːpi］adj. 困倦的

WASH YOUR FACE

对话

Mom：Get up to wash your face.

妈妈：起床洗脸啦。

Philip：Could you help me wash my face?

飞飞：你可以帮我洗脸吗？

Ann：I can wash my face by myself.

安安：我可以自己洗。

Mom：Is it done, sweetie?

妈妈：洗完了吗，亲爱的？

Ann：I'm washing. Could you get me a towel?

安安：我正在洗。可以帮我拿毛巾吗？

Susan：Watch out for the slippery floor, children.

素琴：小心地板滑，孩子们。

词汇

towel ［ˈtaʊəl］n. 毛巾
slippery ［ˈslɪpəri］adj. 滑的

BRUSH YOUR TEETH

对话

Mom：You should brush your teeth after meal, Phil.

妈妈：你应该在吃完饭后刷牙，飞飞。

Philip：OK, can you squeeze the toothpaste for me?

飞飞：好吧，你能帮我挤牙膏吗？

Mom：Sure. Remember to brush your teeth for three minutes.

妈妈：当然可以，记得刷牙三分钟哦。

Ann：I hate brushing my teeth.

安安：我讨厌刷牙。

Mom：Brush your teeth well, or they will turn black and get cavities.

妈妈：好好刷牙，要不牙齿会变黑，长洞洞。

词汇

toothpaste ['tuːθpeɪst] n. 牙膏

squeeze [skwiːz] v. 挤

cavity ['kævəti] n. （牙齿的）龋洞

GET DRESSED

对话

Mom：Let's get dressed. What do you want to wear today, Ann?

妈妈：穿衣服啦。安安，你今天想穿什么？

Ann：I'd like to wear a dress.

安安：我想穿裙子。

Mom：It's a nice day to wear a dress. Do you want to dress yourself?

妈妈：是个穿裙子的好天气。你想自己穿吗？

Ann：I can do it.

安安：我可以。

Susan：You buttoned your dress wrong. Let me help you.

素琴：你的扣子扣错了，我来帮你吧。

Mom：You look great in this dress, sweetie.

妈妈：你穿这条裙子很好看，亲爱的。

词汇

dress [dres] n. 连衣裙；v. 穿衣

button ['bʌtn] v. 扣扣子

weather ['weðə(r)] n. 天气

INSIDE OUT

对话

Mom：Get changed by yourself, Ann.

妈妈：自己换衣服吧，安安。

Ann：Can I wear this?

安安：我可以穿这个吗？

Mom：No, you need to wear your school uniform today.

妈妈：不，你今天要穿校服。

Ann：All right.

安安：好吧。

Mom：You put on your T-shirt inside-out. Let me help you.

妈妈：你的 T 恤里外穿反了。我来帮你吧。

Ann：No. I can do it by myself. I'm a big girl.

安安：不。我自己能行，我是大姑娘了。

词汇

uniform ['juːnɪfɔːm] n. 制服

inside-out 里面朝外

COMB YOUR HAIR

对话

Susan：Let's comb your hair, Ann. I will tie your hair pretty.

素琴：我们来梳头吧，安安。我会给

你扎个漂亮的发型。

Ann：Don't tie it too hard, please.
安安：请不要扎得太紧。

Susan：Sure, do you want a ponytail?
素琴：好的，你想要梳马尾辫吗？

Ann：Yes, I like ponytails.
安安：是的，我喜欢马尾辫。

Susan：Do you want a hairpin?
素琴：你想要别个发卡吗？

Ann：Yes, thank you.
安安：好呀，谢谢。

Ann：I like this hairstyle, thank you.
安安：我喜欢这个发型，谢谢你。

词汇

comb [kəʊm] vt. 梳头发
ponytail [ˈpəʊniteɪl] n. 马尾辫
hairpin [ˈheəpɪn] n. 发卡
hairstyle [ˈheəstaɪl] n. 发型

GO TO THE BATHROOM

对话

Philip：I have to pee.
飞飞：我要尿尿。

Mom：It looks like you are in a rush. Take off your pants first.
妈妈：你看起来很着急，先脱掉裤子。

Philip：Mom, I need you to come!
飞飞：妈妈，我需要你来一下。

Mom：Did you pee in your pants? Don't hold your water next time.

妈妈：你是尿裤子了吗？下次不要憋尿了。

Philip：Sorry. I won't do that again.
飞飞：对不起。我不会再这样了。

Ann：I have to poop.
安安：我要拉便便。

Mom：Don't forget to flush.
妈妈：不要忘记冲厕所。

Ann：It stinks!
安安：好臭呀！

Mom：Remember to wash your hands after pooping.
妈妈：拉完便便记得洗手哦。

Ann：I'm done. Can you help me wipe my bottom?
安安：我拉完了，能帮我擦屁股吗？

词汇

pee [piː] vi. 撒尿
poop [puːp] vi. 排便
flush [flʌʃ] v. 冲掉
stink [stɪŋk] vi. 发恶臭
wipe [waɪp] v. 擦干净
bottom [ˈbɒtəm] n. 臀部

GET READY FOR SCHOOL

对话

Mom：Have you packed your bag? Did you put your homework in your bag?
妈妈：你装好书包了吗？作业放进去了吗？

Ann：Oops, I forgot about my homework.

安安：啊，我忘了装作业。

Mom：You should pack your bag in advance.
妈妈：你应该提前收拾好你的书包。

Ann：I get it.
安安：我明天会都准备好的。

Mom：Hurry up, honey. You will be late.
妈妈：快点，宝贝。你要迟到了。

Ann：Hold on, mom.
安安：我们知道了，妈妈。

Mom：You don't have enough time. Finish packing on the count of three.
妈妈：你的时间不够了，我数到三你要收拾好。

Ann：I'm doing my best.
安安：我正在尽全力。

词汇

pack ［pæk］v. 收拾
in advance 预先

SCHOOL IS OVER

对话

Mom：Honey, Mom is here!
妈妈：宝贝，妈妈在这里！

Ann：Hi, Mom!
安安：嗨，妈妈！

Mom：How was your day?
妈妈：你今天过得怎么样？

Ann：I made a new friend. I want to play with her after school tomorrow.

安安：我交了新朋友。明天放学我想和她一起玩。

Mom：That's good. What did you learn at school?
妈妈：那真好。你今天在学校学了什么呢？

Ann：I had math, science, and painting class today.
安安：我今天上了数学、科学和绘画课。

Mom：Do you like school?
妈妈：你喜欢上学吗？

Ann：Yes, I like school.
安安：是的，我喜欢上学。

词汇

math ［mæθ］n. 数学
science ［ˈsaɪəns］n. 科学
painting ［ˈpeɪntɪŋ］n. 绘画

CLOSE THE DOOR

对话

Mom：Phil, could you close the door for me?
妈妈：飞飞，能帮我把门关上吗？

Philip：Ann, Mom said shut the door.
飞飞：安安，妈妈说把门关上。

Ann：Mom asked you to close the door.
安安：妈妈让你去关门。
(Peng!)
(嘭!)

Mom：Don't slam the door. Close the door gently.

妈妈：不要用力摔门，轻轻地把门关上。

Philip：I got it. I'll be gentle next time.

飞飞：知道了，我下次轻轻地。

词汇

shut〔ʃʌt〕v. 关上
slam〔slæm〕v. 砰地关上
gently〔'dʒentli〕adv. 轻轻地

WATCH TV

对话

Mom：What programme should we watch tonight?

妈妈：今天晚上我们看什么节目呀？

Philip：I want to watch *SpongeBob*.

飞飞：我想看《海绵宝宝》。

Ann：I want to watch *The Octonauts*.

安安：我想看《海底小纵队》。

Mom：Why don't we watch *Peppa Pig* together?

妈妈：要不我们一起看《小猪佩奇》吧。

Philip：I love *Peppa Pig*.

飞飞：我喜欢《小猪佩奇》。

Ann：Me too.

安安：我也喜欢。

Mom：Children, remember to sit back and keep a certain distance from the TV screen.

妈妈：孩子们，记得靠后坐，离电视屏幕保持一定的距离。

Philip：Will you turn down the volume? It's very loud.

飞飞：你能把音量调小吗？非常吵。

Mom：OK.

妈妈：好的。

词汇

programme〔'prəʊɡræm〕n. 节目
volume〔'vɒljuːm〕n. 音量

DON'T PLAY WITH SCISSORS

对话

Philip：Susan could you play paper cutting with me?

飞飞：素琴你能陪我剪纸吗？

Susan：No, Phil, you're too young to play with scissors. It's dangerous.

素琴：不，飞飞，你太小了还不能玩剪刀。太危险了。

Philip：Why?

飞飞：为什么呢？

Susan：Because the scissors are too sharp and it's easy to scratch you.

素琴：因为剪刀太锋利，容易划伤你。

Philip：Well, can you cut out a bunny shape for me?

飞飞：那好吧，你能帮我剪个小兔子吗？

29

Susan：Of course. Bunny is here.
素琴：没问题。小兔子有啦。

词汇

sharp ［ʃɑːp］ adj. 锋利的
scratch ［skrætʃ］ v. 划破
bunny ［ˈbʌni］ n. 兔子（特别是小兔子）

TAKE A BATH

对话

Susan：It's time for a bath.
素琴：该洗澡了哦。

Ann：I want to have a bubble bath.
安安：我想要洗泡泡澡。

Susan：OK, this is your favorite bubble bath. Take off your clothes.
素琴：好的，这是你最喜欢的泡泡澡，脱掉衣服吧。

Ann：I'm going into the tub.
安安：我要进浴缸了。

Susan：Is the water temperature OK?
素琴：水温可以吗？

Ann：It's very comfortable. Look! I've got soap bubbles on my body.
安安：很舒服。看！我身上都是肥皂泡。

Susan：Take a good bath with the soap foam.
素琴：用这些肥皂泡好好洗澡吧。

Ann：Can I play in the tub a little longer?
安安：我能在浴缸多玩一会吗？

Susan：The water is getting cold. Let's wash off the foam now.
素琴：水要凉了，我们把泡泡冲掉吧。

Susan：It's done. Let's dry you with a towel.
素琴：好了，用毛巾给你擦干吧。

Ann：I feel fresh.
安安：我觉得很清爽。

Susan：Be careful! The floor's slippery.
素琴：小心，地板滑。

词汇

bath ［bɑːθ］ n. 沐浴
bubble ［ˈbʌbl］ n. 肥皂泡

WASH YOUR HAIR

对话

Ann：My head is itchy.
安安：我头好痒。

Susan：Your hair smells. Let's wash it.
素琴：你头发臭臭的，来洗头吧。

Ann：I want Mom to help me wash my hair.
安安：我想要妈妈帮我洗头。

Mom：All right. Let's make some foam with the shampoo. Close your eyes or the shampoo will get in your eyes, and it stings.
妈妈：好吧，我们先把头发弄湿，把洗发水搓出泡泡来。闭上眼睛。要不洗发水进了眼睛会痛哦。

Mom：Let's rinse your hair now.
妈妈：现在把头发冲干净吧。

Mom：It's done. Let's wipe your hair with a towel then dry it with a hair dryer.
妈妈：洗完啦，我们用毛巾擦擦，再用吹风机吹干头发。

Ann：I don't want to dry my hair.
安安：我不想吹干头发。

Mom：You will get sick, if you sleep with your hair wet.
妈妈：头发湿着睡觉会生病哦。

词汇

itchy ［ˈɪtʃi］ adj. 发痒的
smell ［smel］ vi. 有难闻的气味
shampoo ［ʃæmˈpuː］ n. 洗发精
sting ［stɪŋ］ v. 刺痛
rinse ［rɪns］ v. 冲洗

PUT ON SOME LOTION

对话

Mom：Let's put on some lotion.
妈妈：我们来擦护肤乳吧。

Ann：Can you put some on my hand? I can put it on by myself.
安安：你可以挤一点在我手上吗？我可以自己抹。

Mom：Be careful not to get any lotion in your eyes.
妈妈：小心不要让护肤乳跑进眼睛。

Ann：OK.
安安：好的。

Mom：How does it feel?
妈妈：感觉如何？

Ann：It's slippery and soft.
安安：滑滑软软的。

Mom：The lotion keeps your skin moist and soft while also keeping it from drying out.
妈妈：护肤乳让你的皮肤水嫩柔软，同时防止它干燥。

Ann：And I smell good now.
安安：我现在闻起来也香香的。

词汇

lotion ［ˈləʊʃn］ n. 护肤乳
moist ［mɔɪst］ adj. 湿润的

DO THE LAUNDRY

对话

Susan：I'm going to do the laundry.
素琴：我要去洗衣服啦。

Ann：I want to help you.
安安：我想给你帮忙。

Susan：OK, put the colored clothes here and the whites over there.
素琴：好呀，帮我把彩色的衣服放在这里，白色的衣服放在那里。

Ann：Gosh! Dad's socks smell bad!
安安：啊！爸爸的袜子好臭！

Susan：Well, let's put the laundry in the washing machine.
素琴：好啦，把要洗的衣服放进洗衣机吧。

Ann：There is a lot of laundry.
安安：有好多衣服要洗。

Susan：Don't put those clothes in the machine. Those clothes need dry-clean.
素琴：不要把那些衣服放进洗衣机。那些衣服得干洗。

词汇

laundry ['lɔːndri] n. 洗衣物的活；要洗的衣服

machine [mə'ʃiːn] n. 机器

HANG UP THE LAUNDRY

对话

Ann：The laundry is done, Mom. Let me help you hang up the clothes.
安安：衣服洗完了，妈妈，我想要帮你晾衣服。

Mom：All right. Put this shirt on the hanger. Make sure the clothes don't hit the floor.
妈妈：好呀，把衬衫挂在衣架上。不要让衣服碰到地板。

Ann：Where do I hang the socks?
安安：袜子晾在哪里？

Mom：Put them on the drying rack.
妈妈：晾在晾衣架上。

Mom：It will be all dry tomorrow.
妈妈：到明天衣服就都干啦。

词汇

hang [hæŋ] v. 悬挂

hanger ['hæŋə(r)] n. 衣架
rack [ræk] n. 架子

GO TO BED

对话

Mom：It's time to go to bed.
妈妈：到睡觉的时间了。

Ann：Mom, I'm not tired yet.
安安：妈妈，我还不困。

Mom：It's over 10 o'clock. You should go to bed, You have to go to school tomorrow.
妈妈：已经10点多了，你该上床睡觉了，明天还要上学。

Ann：OK, Mom. Can you read me a story？
安安：好的，妈妈。能讲个故事给我听吗？

Mom：Sure. Don't forget to go to the bathroom before you go to bed.
妈妈：好的。别忘记睡觉前去洗手间。

Ann：I've already peed.
安安：我已经尿过了。

Mom：Give Mommy a goodnight kiss.
妈妈：给妈妈一个晚安吻。

Ann：Good night, Mom.
安安：晚安，妈妈。

词汇

bathroom ['bɑːθruːm] n. 洗手间

interesting [ˈɪntrəstɪŋ] adj. 有趣的

BEDTIME STORY

对话

 Ann：Mommy, could you read me a story before going to bed?
安安：妈妈，你能在睡觉前给我讲个故事吗?

 Mom：Which story would you like today?
妈妈：今天想听哪个故事呢?

 Ann：I want this one.
安安：我想听这个。

 Mom：You picked a good one. Listen carefully.
妈妈：你选的这个很好，仔细听哦。

 Ann：It's an interesting story. Read one more story for me, Mom.
安安：这个故事真有趣，妈妈，再讲一个。

 Mom：I'll read you one more story. Listen with your eyes closed.
妈妈：我再讲一个故事。闭上眼睛听吧。

 Ann：I'm sleepy.
安安：我想睡了。

 Mom：You can sleep if you feel sleepy.
妈妈：想睡的话就睡吧。

词汇

bedtime [ˈbedtaɪm] n. 就寝时间
pick [pɪk] vt. 选择
carefully [ˈkeəfəli] adv. 小心地

CAN'T FALL ASLEEP

对话

 Ann：Mom, I couldn't fall asleep.
安安：妈妈，我睡不着。

 Mom：Shh, your little brother is already asleep.
妈妈：嘘，弟弟已经睡着了呢。

 Ann：But, I can't fall asleep. I feel a little hungry.
安安：可是，我睡不着。我有点饿了。

 Mom：How about a bottle of warm milk?
妈妈：来杯热牛奶好吗?

 Ann：Thank you, Mom.
安安：谢谢妈妈。

 Mom：Here is your milk. Drink it up. Mom will stay with you until you fall asleep, sweetie.
妈妈：给你热牛奶，都喝完吧。妈妈会陪着你直到你睡着的，亲爱的。

 Ann：I want to sleep with my teddy bear.
安安：我想和我的泰迪熊一起睡。

 Mom：Here you are. I'll put it beside you. Good night, Ann.
妈妈，给你。我把它放在你旁边。晚安，安安。

 Ann：Good night, Mommy.
安安：晚安，妈妈。

词汇

shh ［ʃ］ int. 嘘

beside ［bɪˈsaɪd］ prep. 在旁边

NIGHTMARE

对话

Mom：What's wrong, honey?
妈妈：宝贝，你怎么了？

Ann：Mom, I had a nightmare.
安安：妈妈，我做了个噩梦。

Mom：That wasn't real. It was just a dream.
妈妈：那不是真的，只是个梦。

Ann：It's so dark when I woke up, and I was scared.
安安：我醒来时好黑，我好害怕。

Mom：You're okay now. Mommy's right here.
妈妈：你现在没事了，妈妈就在这里。

Ann：Can you sleep with me tonight, Mom?
安安：妈妈，你今晚能跟我一起睡吗？

Mom：I will sleep next to you. Go back and try to sleep now. Mom will sing you a lullaby.
妈妈：我就睡在你旁边。回去睡觉吧。妈妈唱摇篮曲给你听。

词汇

nightmare ［ˈnaɪtmeə(r)］ n. 噩梦

lullaby ［ˈlʌləbaɪ］ n. 摇篮曲

HAVE A HAIRCUT

对话

Mom：Your hair is too long. You need a haircut.
妈妈：你头发太长了，你需要去剪头发。

Ann：But I like long hair.
安安：可是我喜欢长头发。

Mom：Let's go to a barber shop. Just get it trimmed a little. It won't be too short.
妈妈：我们去理发店吧。稍微修剪一下，不会太短的。

Ann：Alright, I want a beautiful princess hair style.
安安：好吧，我想要个漂亮的公主发型。

词汇

haircut ［ˈheəkʌt］ n. 理发

trim ［trɪm］ v. 修剪

LOOK IN THE MIRROR

对话

Susan：Who is the baby in red? It's Phil.
素琴：这个穿着红色衣服的宝宝是谁呀？这是飞飞。

Susan：These are baby's hands. Let's wave your hands.

素琴：这是宝宝的小手，挥挥小手。

Susan：These are baby's little feet. Let's kick your feet.
素琴：这是宝宝的小脚，我们踢踢小脚。

Susan：This is baby's face. Let's touch your face.
素琴：这是宝宝的小脸，摸摸小脸。

Susan：This is baby's little nose. Let's touch your nose.
素琴：这是宝宝的小鼻子，点点小鼻子。

Susan：These are baby's eye, ear and mouth.
素琴：这是宝宝的眼睛，耳朵和嘴。

词汇

kick ［kɪk］ v. 踢

CHAPTER THREE   INDOOR GAMES

DOWN BY THE STATION

对话

Susan：Welcome to board the train. This train departs from toe station and is bound for finger station.
素琴：欢迎登上火车。这列火车从脚趾站开出，开往手指站。

Susan：Get going from toe now, chug chug, toot toot, reach the knee.
素琴：我们从脚趾出发了，咔嚓咔嚓，嘟嘟，到达膝盖。

Philip：Chug chug, toot toot.
飞飞：咔嚓咔嚓，嘟嘟。

Susan：What's the next station?
素琴：下一站是？

Philip：The tummy. Chug chug, toot toot.
飞飞：肚子。咔嚓咔嚓，嘟嘟。

Susan：Yes, it's the tummy, tickle tickle.
素琴：是的，是肚子，挠痒痒。

Philip：Hah hah, the little train should be serious.
飞飞：哈哈，小火车应该严肃些。

Susan：OK, toot toot. The chest. Chug chug, toot toot, the head. I need to make a U turn.
素琴：好的，嘟嘟。胸部。咔嚓咔嚓，嘟嘟，头。我需要掉头。

Philip：Chug chug, toot toot.
飞飞：咔嚓咔嚓，嘟嘟。

Susan：The shoulder. The train needs to change track. Please extend your arm.
素琴：肩膀。小火车需要变道了。请伸展手臂。

Philip：Done.
飞飞：完成。

Susan：Chug chug, toot toot. What's the name of this railway station?
素琴：咔嚓咔嚓，嘟嘟。这一站的名字是什么？

Philip：Elbow.
飞飞：肘部。

Susan：Chug chug, toot toot, the finger, terminal station. Thank you for traveling.
素琴：咔嚓咔嚓，嘟嘟，手指，终点站。谢谢乘坐。

Philip：It's a pleasant trip.
飞飞：这是一次愉快的旅行。

词汇

elbow ［ˈelbəʊ］ n. 肘部
tummy ［ˈtʌmi］ n. 肚子
track ［træk］ n. 轨道

extend [ɪk'stend] vt. 伸展
terminal ['tɜːmɪnl] n. 终点站

TRAFFIC LIGHTS

对话

 Susan：Phil, do you know what colour it is?
素琴：飞飞，这是什么颜色？

Philip：Red.
飞飞：红色。

Susan：What color is it?
素琴：这是什么颜色？

Philip：Green.
飞飞：绿色。

Susan：What about this one?
素琴：那这个呢？

Philip：Yellow.
飞飞：黄色。

Susan：Now let's play a game called Traffic Lights. Well, listen carefully. The rules of the game are coming. The red light means stop. The green light means go. The yellow light means wait. So, When you see the red light, you have to…
素琴：现在我们玩儿一个交通信号灯的游戏。注意听好，游戏规则来了，红灯停，绿灯行，黄灯亮了等一等。所以当你看到红灯时，你必须……

Philip：Stop.
飞飞：停下。

 Susan：When you see the yellow one, you have to…
素琴：当你看到黄灯，你必须……

 Philip：Wait.
飞飞：等一等。

 Susan：When you see the green one, you can…
素琴：当你看到绿灯，你可以……

 Philip：Go.
飞飞：走。

 Susan：Well, you got the rules, let's get started.
素琴：很好，你掌握了游戏规则，让我们开始游戏吧。

词汇

traffic light　交通灯
mean [miːn] v.　表示……的意思

TAKE A BUS

对话

 Susan：Sitting on my lap, like sitting on a bus. Let's sway to the music.
素琴：坐在我的腿上就像坐在公交车上一样。让我们随着音乐摇摆。
The wheels on the bus go round and round. Round and round.
公交车的车轮转啊转，转啊转。
All through the town.
一路经过城镇。
The horn on the bus goes beep beep beep, beep beep beep.
公交车的喇叭哗哗哗，哗哗哗。
All through the town.

一路经过城镇。

The people on the bus go up and down, up and down.

公交车上的人上上下下，上上下下。

All through the town.

一路经过城镇。

The wipers on the bus go swish left and right, left and right.

公交车的雨刷左左右右，左左右右。

All through the town.

一路经过城镇。

The door on the bus goes open and shut, open and shut.

公交车的门开了关，开了关。

All through the town.

一路经过城镇。

The Driver on the bus says "Move on back", "Move on back".

公交车的司机说"往后走""往后走"。

All through the town.

一路经过城镇。

The babies on the bus go "Wah wah wah", "Wah wah wah".

公交车上的宝宝，哇哇哇哭，哇哇哇哭。

The mommy on the bus shh shh shh.

公交车上的妈妈说嘘嘘嘘。

All through the town.

一路经过城镇。

词汇

lap［læp］n.（坐着时的）大腿部

sway［sweɪ］v. 摇摆

CATCH

对话

Susan：Phil, let's play catch. Are you ready?

素琴：飞飞，我们一起玩儿接球游戏吧，你准备好了吗？

Philip：Yes, I'm ready.

飞飞：准备好了。

Susan：Catch it. I'm going to throw the ball. Great! You caught it. Throw it hard. Whoops, I missed it. The second round is on. Get ready to catch the ball.

素琴：接住哦，我要抛球了，太棒了！你接住了，用力扔。哎哟，我没接住。第二轮开始了，准备接球吧。

Philip：Come on.

飞飞：来吧。

Susan：Oh, no. Keep trying. One more time. Nice catch.

素琴：哦，没接住。继续努力。再来一次。接得好。

Grandma：Can I join in?

姥姥：我能加入吗？

Philip：Let me see. OK, we can form a triangle. I throw the ball to Susan, Susan to Grandma, and Grandma to me.

飞飞：让我想想。可以，我们可以排列成一个三角形，我把球扔给素琴，素琴扔给姥姥，姥姥扔给我。

Susan：What a brilliant idea!
素琴：真是一个好主意！

词汇

form [fɔ:m] v. 排列成
triangle [ˈtraɪæŋgl] n. 三角形
brilliant [ˈbrɪliənt] adj. 非常好的

FINGER DANCE

对话

Susan：Let's draw a father on your thumb.
素琴：我们在大拇指上画个爸爸。

Philip：Dad has short hair.
飞飞：爸爸的头发短短的。

Susan：Draw a Mom on your index finger.
素琴：画个妈妈在食指上。

Philip：Long hair, red lips, Mom is pretty.
飞飞：长长的头发，红红的嘴唇，妈妈很漂亮。

Susan：Yes, Mom is pretty. Sister on the middle finger. She has big eyes and a small mouth.
素琴：是的，妈妈很漂亮。姐姐画在中指，她有大大的眼睛和小小的嘴巴。

Philip：And a braid.
飞飞：还有个辫子。

Susan：Brother on the ring finger. Baby on pinkie. Let's start singing *Finger Family*. The fingers need to dance to it.

素琴：无名指是哥哥。小拇指是宝宝。我们开始唱《手指家庭》了，手指们也要跟着跳舞。

Susan：Daddy Finger, Daddy Finger, where are you?
素琴：手指爸爸，手指爸爸，你在哪儿？

Philip：Here I am! Here I am.
飞飞：我在这里，我在这里

Susan：How are you, today?
素琴：今天怎么样？

Philip：Very well, thank you.
飞飞：很好，谢谢你。

Susan：Mommy Finger, Mommy Finger, where are you?
素琴：手指妈妈，手指妈妈，你在哪儿？

Philip：Here I am! Here I am.
飞飞：我在这里！我在这里。

Susan：How are you, today?
素琴：你今天怎么样？

Philip：Very well, thank you.
飞飞：很好，谢谢你。

Susan：Brother Finger, Brother Finger, where are you?
素琴：手指哥哥，手指哥哥，你在哪儿？

Philip：Here I am! Here I am.
飞飞：我在这里！我在这里。

Susan：How are you, today?
素琴：你今天怎么样？

Philip：Very well, thank you.
飞飞：很好，谢谢你。

词汇

thumb［θʌm］n. 拇指
index finger　食指
middle finger　中指
ring finger　无名指
braid［breɪd］n. 辫子
pinkie［ˈpɪŋki］n. 小拇指

GUESS WHO I AM

对话

Susan：Woof woof, guess who I am?
素琴：汪汪，猜猜我是谁？

Philip：Dog.
飞飞：狗狗。

Susan：You are so smart.
素琴：你真聪明。

Susan：Quack quack quack, guess who I am.
素琴：嘎嘎嘎，猜猜我是谁？

Philip：Duckling?
飞飞：小鸭子？

Susan：That's right. Let me guess who you are?
素琴：猜对了。让我猜猜你是谁？

Philip：Meow meow.
飞飞：喵喵。

Susan：Kitten.
素琴：小猫。

Philip：Clever Susan.
飞飞：聪明的素琴。

Susan：I am round and red. It tastes sweet and crunchy. I am a kind of fruit.
素琴：我又圆又红，吃起来甜甜的，脆脆的。我是一种水果。

Philip：Apple?
飞飞：苹果？

Susan：Right. I am brown. I have warm soft fur. I am tall and strong. I like to eat sweet honey. Who am I?
素琴：正确。我是棕色的，我有暖暖的软软的毛，我长得高高大大的，我喜欢吃甜甜的蜂蜜，我是谁？

Philip：Bear?
飞飞：熊？

Susan：You guessed it again. Another one, I can swim. I live in the water. I have four legs. Wearing green clothes. Please guess who I am?
素琴：你又猜中了。再来一个，我会游泳，我生活在水里。我有四只脚，穿着绿衣服。请你猜猜我是谁？

Philip：I don't know.
飞飞：不知道。

Susan：I am the tadpole's mother.
素琴：我是小蝌蚪的妈妈。

Philip：Frog?
飞飞：青蛙？

Susan：Great, you're right. I have a big pocket with my baby in it. I am good at jumping.
素琴：很棒，你答对了。我有一个大口袋，里边装着我的小宝贝，我擅长跳跃。

Philip：Kangaroo.

飞飞：袋鼠。

Susan：Excellent！

素琴：非常棒！

词汇

duckling［ˈdʌklɪŋ］n. 小鸭子

kitten［ˈkɪtn］n. 小猫

crunchy［ˈkrʌntʃi］adj. 脆的

tadpole［ˈtædpəʊl］n. 蝌蚪

ROLLER COASTER BY DAD

对话

Dad：Would you like to get on a roller coaster?

爸爸：你想坐过山车吗？

Philip：Sure. Are we going to the playground?

飞飞：当然，我们要去游乐场吗？

Dad：The roller coaster that I talked about is a game. And, we will play at home.

爸爸：我说的过山车是一个游戏。我们在家里玩儿。

Philip：How to play?

飞飞：怎样玩儿？

Dad：Face to me. I will put my hands under your arms from your back to hold you. Are you ready? The roller coaster is setting off.

爸爸：你面向我。我从后背把手伸到你的腋下抓住你。你准备好了吗？过山车出发喽。

Philip：I'm ready.

飞飞：我准备好了。

Dad：Once, twice, three times. I'm so tired that I need a rest.

爸爸：一圈，两圈，三圈。我太累了，我要休息。

Philip：This game is so exciting.

飞飞：这个游戏好刺激。

词汇

roller coaster　过山车

SLIDE BY DAD

对话

Dad：I'm a slide. Who wants to play with me?

爸爸：我是滑梯，谁想和我玩儿呢？

Philip：I want to play.

飞飞：我想玩儿。

Dad：OK, Come here, sit on my lap. I will put my hands under your arms to hold you.

爸爸：好的，过来，坐在我的腿上。我要把我的双手放在你的腋下扶住你。

Dad：I need a helper. Who want to help?

爸爸：我需要一个助手，谁想帮忙？

Susan：I'll be your helper. What should I do?

素琴：我来做你的助手，我需要做什么呢？

Dad：Keep him safe as he slides down.

爸爸：在他滑下去的时候，保护他的安全。

 Susan：OK.

素琴：好的。

 Dad：Are you ready, Phil?

爸爸：飞飞准备好了吗？

 Philip：Yes, hurry up.

飞飞：是的，快点儿吧。

 Dad：Watch out, I'll push you down.

爸爸：当心，我要推你下去了。

 Philip：It's so much fun. I want to play one more time.

飞飞：太有意思了，我还想再玩儿一次。

词汇

hurry ['hʌri] v. 赶快

slide [slaɪd] n. 滑梯；v. 滑行

DAD IS AN APPLE TREE

对话

 Dad：Could you do me a favour, please?

爸爸：你能帮我一个忙吗？

 Philip：What can I do?

飞飞：我能做什么？

 Dad：Can you get me several red ocean balls? I will stick them on my body.

爸爸：你能给我找一些红色的海洋球吗？我要把这些球贴到身上。

 Philip：OK.

飞飞：可以。

 Dad：Oh, I also need a roll of double-sided tape.

爸爸：我还需要一卷双面胶。

 Philip：What do you want to do, daddy?

飞飞：爸爸你想做什么？

 Dad：It's a secret, but you will get the answer in a minute.

爸爸：这是一个秘密，但是你很快就会知道了。

 Dad：Look at me. I am a tall apple tree. I have many red apples. They are crunchy and sweet. Does anyone want to climb and pick the apples? Oh, there is a naughty little boy. Would you like an apple?

爸爸：快看我，我是一棵高高的苹果树，我有很多的红苹果，他们又脆又甜。有人想要爬上来摘苹果吗？哦，这里有一个淘气的小男孩，请问你想要红苹果吗？

 Philip：Yes, I like apples.

飞飞：是的，我喜欢苹果。

 Dad：Try to climb up the tree and pick them.

爸爸：努力爬上树摘苹果吧。

 Philip：I'm coming.

飞飞：我来了。

 Dad：Come on. You're getting closer to these apples.

爸爸：加油，你离苹果越来越近了。

 Dad：Well, you got an apple, I still have four left.

爸爸：很好，你摘到了一个苹果，我还有四个。

Philip: I'll pick up all your apples.
飞飞：我要摘光所有的苹果。

Dad: Congratulations on achieving your goal. You've picked all the apples on your own.
爸爸：祝贺你目标达成，你自己摘到了所有的苹果。

Dad: You can wash it and have a taste. Does it taste good?
爸爸：你可以洗一洗，尝一尝，这个苹果好吃吗？

Philip: Yes.
飞飞：是的。

词汇

favour [ˈfeɪvə(r)] n. 帮助
double – sided tape　双面胶带
naughty [ˈnɔːti] adj. 淘气的
achieve [əˈtʃiːv] vt. 达到
pick [pɪk] vt. 采；摘

COGNITIVE EXERCISE

对话

Susan: Phil, look at the picture, what is this?
素琴：飞飞，看图片上的是什么？

Susan: This is an apple, apple, red apple, sweet apple.
素琴：这是苹果，苹果，红色的苹果，甜甜的苹果。

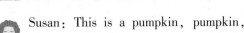
Susan: This is a lemon, lemon, yellow lemon, sour lemon.
素琴：这是柠檬，柠檬，黄色的柠檬，酸酸的柠檬。

Susan: This is a watermelon, watermelon, green watermelon, sweet watermelon.
素琴：这是西瓜，西瓜，绿色的西瓜，甜甜的西瓜。

Susan: They are fruits.
素琴：它们是水果。

Susan: This is a pumpkin, pumpkin, orange pumpkin, round pumpkin.
素琴：这是南瓜，南瓜，橘色的南瓜，圆圆的南瓜。

Susan: This is a pepper, pepper, red pepper, hot pepper.
素琴：这是辣椒，辣椒，红色的辣椒，辣辣的辣椒。

Susan: They are vegetables.
素琴：它们是蔬菜。

词汇

pumpkin [ˈpʌmpkɪn] n. 南瓜
pepper [ˈpepə(r)] n. 辣椒
projector [prəˈdʒektə(r)] n. 投影仪

I'M AN AIRPLANE

对话

Dad: Do you want to play a game of flying?
爸爸：你想玩儿飞行游戏么？

Philip: Yes.
飞飞：是的。

Dad: You need to lay on your stomach on my shins. Little plane, are you ready to take off?

爸爸：你要趴在我的小腿上。小飞机，你准备好起飞了吗？

Philip：Yes.

飞飞：是的。

Dad：Okay, The plane is taking off. Keep balance.

爸爸：好的，小飞机起飞喽。保持平衡。

Philip：Susan, come on!

飞飞：素琴，快来啊!

Susan：What are you doing?

素琴：你们在干什么？

Philip：I'm flying, it's so interesting.

飞飞：我正在飞，太有趣了。

词汇

shin [ʃɪn] n. 胫骨

BUILD BLOCKS

对话

Susan：Let's play with the blocks. This is red. Red.

素琴：我们来玩积木吧。这是红色的。

Philip：Red.

飞飞：红色。

Susan：Phil, can you tell me what color is it?

素琴：飞飞，你能告诉我这是什么颜色吗？

Philip：Red.

飞飞：红色。

Susan：Could you get me a red block, please? Look, I built a tall building.

素琴：请你帮我拿一块红色的积木好吗？快看我搭了一座高楼。

Susan：Oh, you pushed them, so they fell down.

素琴：哦，你推了它们，所以它们倒塌了。

Susan：Since it fell down, let's line up the blocks.

素琴：既然倒塌了，我们就把积木排列起来吧。

Susan：What do you want to build with the blocks?

素琴：你想用积木搭什么？

Philip：I want to build a road roller. Can you help me?

飞飞：我想搭一个压路机，你能帮助我吗？

Susan：Let me see. We need wheels, a chassis, steel wheels and a frame of the roller.

素琴：让我想想。我们需要车轮、车底盘、钢轮和车架。

Philip：Where does the driver sit?

飞飞：司机坐在哪儿？

Susan：Oh, I forgot the cab.

素琴：哦，我忘了驾驶室。

Philip：We also need a chimney.

飞飞：我们还需要一个烟筒。

Susan：It looks great.

素琴：看起来很不错。

词汇

line up　排列起
road roller　压路机
chassis ['ʃæsi] n. 底盘
steel wheel　钢轮
cab [kæb] n. 驾驶室

INDOOR PLAY GROUND

对话

Susan：Phil, we can't go in there unless we take off our shoes and put them on the shoe rack.
素琴：飞飞，我们得把鞋子脱掉，放到鞋架上才能进去。

Philip：There are so many colored balls here. This is red, this is green, this is yellow, this is blue.
飞飞：这里有好多彩色的球。这是红色的，这是绿色的，这是黄色的，这是蓝色的。

Susan：I'll cover you with balls. Now I'm a digger. Dig, dig, dig. I get a child. Who are you?
素琴：我先用球把你盖上。现在我是挖掘机，挖，挖，挖。我挖到一个小朋友。你是谁呀？

Philip：I'm Phil.
飞飞：我是飞飞。

词汇

shoe rack　鞋架
digger ['dɪgə(r)] n. 挖掘机

THE SLIDE

对话

Philip：There's a long slide. I'd like to slide. Can you come with me?
飞飞：这有一个长长的滑梯，我想滑滑梯，你可以陪我一起吗？

Susan：OK, let's go up by the steps and down the slide.
素琴：好的，我们从这个阶梯爬上去，然后从滑梯滑下来。

Susan：Keep your body leaning forward. Are you ready? Let's count one, two, three and let go.
素琴：要保持身体前倾，你准备好了吗，我们数1、2、3，然后出发。

Philip：One, two, three, go.
飞飞：1、2、3，出发。

Susan：One, two, three, go.
素琴：1、2、3，出发。

Philip：I want to play again.
飞飞：想要再玩儿一次。

Susan：OK, go ahead.
素琴：好的，去吧。

词汇

forward ['fɔːwəd] adv. 向前

TRAMPOLINE

对话

Susan：Let's go and play on the trampoline.

素琴：我们去玩儿蹦蹦床吧。

Susan：Bounce, bounce, bounce, bend your knees, keep your balance, make a turn, oh, you fell down. Are you OK?

素琴：弹、弹、弹，膝盖弯曲，保持平衡，转一圈，哦，你摔倒了。你还好吧？

Philip：I'm OK.

飞飞：我很好。

Susan：Let's take a break.

素琴：让我们休息一会儿吧。

Philip：Can you play with me?

飞飞：你可以和我一起玩儿吗？

Susan：Oh no, it's for kids only. I'm too heavy.

素琴：哦，不可以，这只适合小朋友，我太重了。

Susan：Philip, don't lie there. There are a lot of little feet jumping around you. You are easily trampled by other children. Stand up. Go on jumping. If you are tired, come down and have a rest.

素琴：飞飞，不要躺下，有很多小脚丫在你周围跳跃，你容易被别的小朋友踩到。快站起来，我们继续跳。如果你累了，下来休息一下。

词汇

trampoline［ˈtræmpəliːn］n. 蹦床

FOAM BLOCKS

对话

Susan：There are lots of big foam blocks.

素琴：这里有很多大泡沫积木。

Philip：I have a great idea.

飞飞：我有一个好主意。

Susan：What is your idea?

素琴：是什么主意？

Philip：Let's play bowling.

飞飞：我们来玩儿保龄球吧。

Susan：OK, let's learn the shapes before we start playing. This is a cylinder and this is a cuboid.

素琴：好的，我们开始玩之前先认识一下形状。这是圆柱体，这是长方体。

Susan：Phil, we use cylinder blocks as bowling pins. Can you help me find six cylinders?

素琴：飞飞，我们把圆柱体的积木当作保龄球瓶，你能帮我找到6个圆柱体吗？

Philip：OK.

飞飞：好的。

Susan：One, two, three, four, five. We need one more.

素琴：1，2，3，4，5，我们还需要

一个。

Philip：Here you are.
飞飞：给你。

Susan：Let's line them up. Now we need a big ball.
素琴：我们把它们排好。现在我们需要一个大大的球。

Philip：There is a bounce ball.
飞飞：那有一个蹦蹦球。

Susan：Go to get it.
素琴：去拿过来吧。

词汇

bowling ['bəʊlɪŋ] n. 保龄球

ROLE PLAY

对话

Susan：Today, let's play the role of kindergarten kid and teacher. Who will be the teacher first?
素琴：今天我们来扮演幼儿园里的小朋友和老师。谁先当老师？

Philip：Me.
飞飞：我。

Susan：OK. Action.
素琴：好的。开始喽。

Susan：I'm thirsty, can I have some water, Mr. Li?
素琴：我渴了，李老师，我能喝水吗？

Philip：OK, here you are.
飞飞：好的，给你。

Susan：Thank you, Mr. Li.
素琴：谢谢李老师。

Susan：I want to pee, Mr. Li.
素琴：李老师，我想小便。

Philip：Come with me. Let's go to the bathroom.
飞飞：跟我来。我们去卫生间。

Susan：Time to switch roles. Now, I am Ms. Wang.
素琴：该交换角色了。现在，我是王老师。

Philip：Ms. Wang, I want to play with toys.
飞飞：王老师，我想玩儿玩具。

Susan：Please wait for ten minutes. You can play with toys after class.
素琴：请稍等十分钟，下课后你就可以玩儿玩具了。

Philip：I want to draw a picture, Ms. Wang.
飞飞：王老师，我想画画。

Susan：Here are crayons. What color do you like?
素琴：这是蜡笔。你想要什么颜色的？

Philip：I'd like blue, purple, green and orange. Thank you.
飞飞：我想要蓝色的，紫色的，绿色的和橙色的，谢谢。

Susan：You're welcome. What do you want to draw?
素琴：不用谢，你想画什么？

Philip：An excavator.
飞飞：一辆挖掘机。

Susan：You really like engineering trucks.

素琴：你真的好喜欢工程车。

词汇

crayon ［ˈkreɪən］ n. 蜡笔
excavator ［ˈekskəveɪtə(r)］ n. 挖掘机

TAKE CARE OF PLANTS

对话

Susan：Phil, a beautiful sunflower for you. Do you like it?

素琴：飞飞，送你一朵漂亮的向日葵。你喜欢吗？

Philip：Yes, it's yellow. Yellow means happy.

飞飞：喜欢，它是黄色的，黄色代表开心。

Susan：We're going to put it in a vase with some water.

素琴：我们要插到有水的花瓶里。

Philip：Why in the water?

飞飞：为什么要插进水里？

Susan：Will you get thirsty if you don't drink water?

素琴：如果你不喝水会不会口渴？

Philip：I will.

飞飞：会。

Susan：Well, the flower needs water just like Phil. Without water, the flower will soon wither.

素琴：嗯，小花像飞飞一样，也需要喝水，没有水，小花会很快枯萎的。

（A few days later）
（几天后）

Philip：The flower looks terrible.

飞飞：花儿看起来很糟糕。

Susan：Let me see. Oh, it's wilted.

素琴：我看看。喔，它枯萎了。

Philip：Why is this happening?

飞飞：为什么会这样？

Susan：Because they don't have roots to absorb more nutrients.

素琴：因为它们没有根来吸收更多的营养物质。

Philip：I'd like to have a plant with roots.

飞飞：我想要有根的植物。

Susan：Phil, I have a present for you.

素琴：我有礼物送给你。

Philip：What's this?

飞飞：这是什么？

Susan：This is a bag of seeds, we plant the seeds and look after them.

素琴：这是一包种子。我们种下种子并照顾它们。

Philip：What should I do?

飞飞：那要怎么做？

Susan：First we need to plant the seeds in a pot full of soil.

素琴：首先我们把种子种在装满土壤的花盆中。

Philip：This is their home.

飞飞：就是它们的家了。

Susan：Plants need water and sunshine. Place the pot in the sun. You need to water them properly every day. Then wait patiently for them to sprout.

素琴：植物需要水和阳光。把花盆放在阳光下。你要每天给它们浇适量的水，然后耐心等待它们发芽。

(Several days later)

（几天后）

Philip：They have sprouted.

飞飞：它们发芽了。

Susan：Don't forget to water your plants.

素琴：不要忘记给你的植物浇水。

词汇

absorb [əbˈzɔːb] v. 吸收

SIMON SAYS

对话

Susan：Today we're going to play a game, Simon says. If I say "Simon says jump", you jump. If I say "Simon says touch your nose", you touch your nose. But if I don't say "Simon says" first, don't move. Do you get it?

素琴：今天我们玩儿一个游戏：西蒙说。如果我说"西蒙说跳"，你就跳。如果我说"西蒙说摸你的鼻子"，你就摸你的鼻子。如果我说的指令前没有"西蒙说"，就不要动。你明白了吗？

Philip：Yes, I think so.

飞飞：我想是的。

Susan：Let's play the game. Are you ready?

素琴：让我们玩儿游戏吧。你准备好了吗？

Philip：Yes, I'm ready.

飞飞：是的，我准备好了。

Susan：Simon says touch your ear (eyebrow, forehead, jaw, cheek).

素琴：西蒙说摸你的耳朵（眉毛，前额，下巴，脸颊）。

Susan：Squat (clap your hands, sit down, turn around, stamp).

素琴：蹲下（鼓掌，坐下，转身，跺脚）。

Susan：I didn't say "Simon says" first. You shouldn't move.

素琴：我没有说"西蒙说"，你不应该动。

Susan：Simon says raise your left hand (right hand).

素琴：西蒙说举起你的左手（右手）。

Susan：Do you want to take turn to be "Simon"?

素琴：你想当西蒙吗？

Philip：I'd love to. Let's switch roles.

飞飞：我想当。我们交换角色吧。

Susan：OK, give the orders, Simon.

素琴：好的，西蒙发布指令吧。

Philip：Simon says take off your slippers.

飞飞：西蒙说脱掉你的拖鞋。

词汇

eyebrow [ˈaɪbraʊ] n. 眉毛

jaw〔dʒɔ:〕n. 下巴
squat〔skwɒt〕v. 蹲下
stamp〔stæmp〕v. 跺脚
switch〔swɪtʃ〕vt. 交换
slipper〔'slɪpə(r)〕n. 拖鞋

EMOTIONAL GAME

对话

Susan：Phil, let's play an emotional game.
素琴：飞飞，我们玩儿一个情绪游戏吧。

Philip：OK.
飞飞：好的。

Susan：I'm going to perform. Can you guess what mood I'm in?
素琴：我来表演，你能猜出我的心情吗？

Philip：OK.
飞飞：好的。

Susan：Humph!
素琴：哼!

Philip：Angry.
飞飞：生气。

Susan：Haha.
素琴：哈哈。

Philip：Happy.
飞飞：高兴。

Susan：Boohoo.
素琴：呜呜。

Philip：You are crying, you are sad.
飞飞：你在哭，你难过了。

Susan：Now let's look some pictures. What is the expression in this picture?
素琴：现在我们来看一些图片，这张图片里的表情是什么？

Philip：Scared.
飞飞：害怕。

Susan：What about this one?
素琴：这张呢？

Philip：Surprised.
飞飞：惊讶。

Susan：Well, it's time to update the game. What do you do, if you are angry?
素琴：很好，现在要升级游戏了。如果你生气了，你该怎么办？

Philip：Maybe I'll cry.
飞飞：或许我会哭。

Susan：Do you remember how Horace deals with his anger in the book Mean Soup?
素琴：你记得在《生气汤》里，霍瑞斯生气后是怎么做的吗？

Philip：He and his mother made a batch of Mean Soup.
飞飞：他和妈妈做了一锅生气汤。

Susan：Yeah, then they smiled. We need to get our bad feelings out instead of locking them, then we'll feel better. We can also use their method to stir away bad feelings.
素琴：对，然后他们笑了。我们需要把坏的感受表达出来而不是藏起来，这样我们才会开心。我们也可以用他们的方法驱散坏情绪。

词汇

mood [muːd] n. 情绪

expression [ɪkˈspreʃn] n. 表情

deal with 处理

batch [bætʃ] n. 一批

stir [stɜː(r)] v. 搅拌

instead of 代替

PLAY BALL GAMES

对话

Ann：Philip, will you join us to play ball games?

安安：飞飞，你跟我一起玩球吧。

Philip：Sure!

飞飞：好的!

Susan：How do we play?

素琴：我们怎么玩儿呢?

Philip：We can play throw and catch. We can also bounce the ball.

飞飞：我们可以互相抛接球，我们也可以拍球。

Susan：It will disturb the neighbours if we bounce the ball in the room. We can't do that.

素琴：如果我们在房间里拍球会打扰邻居，我们不能那样做。

Ann：Two of us walk with the ball in our arms, then pass the ball to the other.

安安：我们两个人一起抱球走，然后把球传给另一个人。

Susan：Good idea, Ann. Let's play together.

素琴：好主意，安安。我们一起玩儿吧。

词汇

bounce [baʊns] v. 使弹起

neighbour [ˈneɪbə(r)] n. 邻居

READ PICTURE BOOKS

对话

Ann：Read us a story, Mom.

安安：妈妈，给我们讲个故事吧。

Mom：Which book do you want to read?

妈妈：你们想读哪一本?

Philip：*Feeding Time.*

飞飞：《喂食时间》。

Mom：OK, let's read together. What does the breeder feed the polar bear?

妈妈：好的，我们一起看，饲养员喂了北极熊什么?

Ann：Fish.

安安：鱼。

Mom：What about the penguin?

妈妈：企鹅呢?

Philip：Fish too.

飞飞：也是鱼。

Mom：What do dolphins and whales eat?

妈妈：海豚和鲸鱼吃什么?

Ann：Fish.

安安：鱼。

Mom：What does Mr. Seal like to eat?
妈妈：海豹先生喜欢吃什么？

Philip：Fish too.
飞飞：也是鱼。

Mom：OK, all of the animal friends in the aquarium have had lunch. What about the breeder?
妈妈：好的，海洋馆的动物朋友们都吃过午饭了，那饲养员呢？

Ann：The breeder goes to lunch.
安安：饲养员也去吃午饭了。

Mom：What does she eat?
妈妈：她在吃什么？

Philip：She is eating fried fish.
飞飞：她在吃炸鱼。

词汇

breeder ［ˈbriːdə(r)］ n. 饲养员

polar bear　北极熊

penguin ［ˈpeŋgwɪn］ n. 企鹅

dolphin ［ˈdɒlfɪn］ n. 海豚

whale ［weɪl］ n. 鲸鱼

seal ［siːl］ n. 海豹

aquarium ［əˈkweəriəm］ n. 海洋馆

MAKE A PAPER AIRPLANE

对话

Philip：Wow, Susan, what a cool paper airplane!
飞飞：哇，素琴，好酷的纸飞机！

Ann：I like this paper airplane.
安安：我喜欢这个纸飞机。

Susan：I'll show you how to make one.
素琴：我教你们怎么折纸飞机。

Philip：Great!
飞飞：太好了！

Ann：Susan, the paper is too big to make one paper plane. I'll have to cut it off with scissors.
安安：素琴，这张纸折一个纸飞机太大。我需要用剪刀剪一下。

Susan：Ann, don't take the big scissors. It is unsafe for you. You should use children's safety scissors.
素琴：安安，不要拿大人的剪刀。这个对你来说不安全。你应该用儿童安全剪刀。

Ann：OK Susan, I'll keep that in mind.
安安：好的素琴，我记住了。

词汇

airplane ［ˈeəpleɪn］ n. 飞机

MAKE LANTERNS

对话

Susan：The Lantern Festival is coming up soon. Would you like to make lanterns with me?
素琴：马上到元宵节了，你愿意跟我一起做彩灯吗？

Ann：I'd love to.
安安：我们愿意。

Philip：I'd love to.
飞飞：我们愿意。

Susan：First of all, let's open the lantern and fix it to the bamboo skeleton, then we will color it.

素琴：首先，把灯笼撑开，固定在竹子骨架上，然后我们要给它涂颜色。

Ann：I'll paint it in pink.

安安：我要涂粉色。

Philip：I'll paint it in blue.

飞飞：我要涂蓝色。

Ann：I also want to paint it in orange.

安安：我还要涂橘色。

Philip：I want to paint it in red.

飞飞：我想涂红色。

Susan：We can paint it in seven colors. One more color for each of you.

素琴：我们可以涂七种颜色。你们每人再涂一种颜色。

Ann：Well, I'd like yellow.

安安：好吧，我要涂黄色。

Philip：I'd like green.

飞飞：我要涂绿色。

Susan：At last, let me do purple. Our seven-color lantern is now complete.

素琴：最后，我来涂紫色。好了，我们的七色彩灯做好了。

Ann：Such a beautiful lantern. It's the color of the rainbow.

安安：好漂亮的灯笼。是彩虹颜色的呢。

词汇

lantern festival　元宵节

bamboo［ˌbæm'buː］n. 竹子

skeleton［'skelɪtn］n. 骨架

GUESSING GAME

对话

Susan：Let's play a guessing game. I'll name a part of an animal's body, and then you guess what animal it is.

素琴：我们来玩儿个猜谜游戏，我说出动物身体的一个部位，然后你们猜猜它是什么动物。

Ann and Philip：OK.

安安，飞飞：好的。

Susan：Black eyes.

素琴：黑眼睛。

Ann：Panda.

安安：熊猫。

Susan：Long neck.

素琴：长脖子。

Philip：Giraffe.

飞飞：长颈鹿。

Susan：Long and sharp mouth.

素琴：长长尖尖的嘴。

Ann：Woodpecker.

安安：啄木鸟。

Susan：Long nose.

素琴：长鼻子。

Philip：Elephant.

飞飞：大象。

Susan：Who has two humps on its back?

素琴：谁的后背有两个驼峰？

Ann：Camel.
安安：骆驼。

Susan：Great. The last one. Whose feather is colorful and spread out like a fan?
素琴：真棒。最后一个。谁的羽毛五颜六色，展开像扇子?

Philip：Parrot.
飞飞：鹦鹉。

Ann：No. It's a peacock.
安安：不对。是孔雀。

Susan：Yes, peacock.
素琴：是的，是孔雀。

词汇

giraffe ［dʒəˈrɑːf］n. 长颈鹿

woodpecker ［ˈwʊdpekə(r)］n. 啄木鸟

camel ［ˈkæml］n. 骆驼

feather ［ˈfeðə(r)］n. 羽毛

spread ［spred］vt. 展开

fan ［fæn］n. 扇子

peacock ［ˈpiːkɒk］n. 孔雀

ASSEMBLE JIGSAW PUZZLES

对话

Philip：What are you doing, Ann?
飞飞：你在做什么，安安?

Ann：I'm playing the jigsaw puzzles.
安安：我正在拼拼图。

Philip：I want to play with you.
飞飞：我想跟你一起玩。

Ann：You're too young to play it. Don't bother me.
安安：你太小了不会玩儿。别打扰我。

Mom：Honey, he might be able to play some simple ones.
妈妈：宝贝，也许他可以拼一些简单的。

Ann：OK.
安安：好吧。

Mom：Philip, do you know what the colour of a zebra is?
妈妈：飞飞，你知道斑马是什么颜色的吗?

Philip：Black and white.
飞飞：黑色和白色。

Mom：That's right. Now you'll try to make a zebra out of the pieces in these colors.
妈妈：对，现在你试着用这些颜色的拼块拼成斑马。

Philip：OK, Mom. Is it right?
飞飞：好的妈妈。这样对吗?

Mom：Good job!
妈妈：非常好!

词汇

jigsaw puzzle 拼图

PLAY LEGO

对话

Ann：Philip, let's play lego together.
安安：飞飞，咱们一起拼乐高吧。

Philip：Great, I want to play the Police Station.

飞飞：好，我想玩"警察局"。

Ann：OK, I'll build the police station. Phil, can you make the police car?

安安：好的，我来拼这个警察局。飞飞，你能拼警车吗？

Philip：It's difficult.

飞飞：好难。

Susan：Phil, would you like to play a simple one, the Digital Train.

素琴：飞飞，你愿意玩这个简单的数字小火车游戏吗？

Philip：Great!

飞飞：太好了！

Susan：Connect the train carriage in a digital order.

素琴：按数字顺序连接火车车厢。

Philip：OK, one, two, three. four, five, six. seven, eight, nine. It's finished.

飞飞：好，1，2，3。4，5，6。7，8，9。我完成了。

Susan：Good job Philip.

素琴：做得好飞飞。

词汇

digital ['dɪdʒɪtl] adj. 数字的

carriage ['kærɪdʒ] n. 车厢

PLAY THE ROCK – PAPER – SCISSORS GAME

对话

Susan：Let's play the Rock – Paper – Scissors game.

素琴：咱们来玩儿石头剪刀布的游戏吧。

Ann，Philip：Great!

安安，飞飞：太好了！

Susan：Rock – Paper – Scissors. Look, two players threw paper. What does it look like?

素琴：石头，剪刀，布。看，两个玩家出了布。这看起来像什么？

Ann：A butterfly.

安安：一只蝴蝶。

Susan：That's right. Rock – Paper – Scissors. Philip won. Look, there's a rock on the top and the paper under it. What does it look like?

素琴：对。石头，剪刀，布。飞飞赢了。看，上面一个石头，下面是布，这看起来像什么？

Philip：A jellyfish.

飞飞：一只水母。

Susan：Philip is so smart. Rock – Paper – Scissors. Ann got it. This time we got a rock on the top and the scissors under it. What does it look like?

素琴：飞飞真聪明。石头，剪刀，布。安安赢了。这次我们有一个石头在上面，一个剪刀在下面，这看起来像什么？

Ann：It's a snail!
安安：是一只蜗牛！

Susan：Great! The last round. Rock – Paper – Scissors. You both threw scissors. Two scissors are together. What does it look like?
素琴：太棒了！最后一轮。石头，剪刀，布。你们都出的剪刀。两把剪刀在一起，这看起来像什么？

Ann：It's a crab!
安安：是螃蟹！

Susan：Excellent!
素琴：非常好！

词汇

butterfly ['bʌtəflaɪ] n. 蝴蝶
jellyfish ['dʒelifɪʃ] n. 水母
snail [sneɪl] n. 蜗牛
crab [kræb] n. 螃蟹

PLAY WITH PLASTICINE

对话

Susan：Look here, kids.
素琴：看这里孩子们。

Ann：Wow, colorful plasticine!
安安：哇，五颜六色的橡皮泥！

Susan：Do you want to make animals with the plasticine?
素琴：要不要用橡皮泥来捏小动物？

Philip：Of course.
飞飞：当然。

Susan：What should we make first?
素琴：我们先捏什么呢？

Ann：A bunny.
安安：小兔子。

Susan：OK, what features does a bunny has?
素琴：好，小兔子有什么特点？

Philip：Long ears and short tail.
飞飞：长耳朵和短尾巴。

Ann：Bunny's eyes are red. The mouth has three petals. The body is white.
安安：兔子的眼睛是红色的。嘴巴有三瓣。身体是白色的。

Susan：That's right. Philip, can you make the bunny's head and ears?
素琴：没错。飞飞，你能做小兔子的头和耳朵吗？

Philip：I can do it.
飞飞：我可以。

Susan：Ann, can you make the bunny's body, tail and four legs?
素琴：安安，你可以做小兔子的身体、尾巴和四条腿吗？

Ann：No problem.
安安：没问题。

Susan：Good, put them together to make a cute bunny. What should you do after playing with plasticine?
素琴：非常好，把它们组合到一起做成可爱的小白兔。玩过橡皮泥之后要做什么？

Ann：Wash hands.
安安：洗手。

Susan：Well，let's wash our hands now.
素琴：好，我们去洗手吧。

词汇

plasticine [ˈplæstəsiːn] n. 橡皮泥
tail [teɪl] n. 尾巴
petal [petl] n. 花瓣

MAKE POTTERY

对话

 Susan：You'll have an art class later. This time，you'll learn how to make pottery with clay.
素琴：一会儿你上美术课。这次课你要学习用陶土做陶器。

 Ann：Wow，it's fantastic！
安安：哇，太棒了！

 Susan：Take a look at the cup. First of all，the clay is molded into a cup-like shape，then it will be colored. Finally，we fire the clay at a high temperature，and get a cup.
素琴：看看这个杯子。首先，用陶土塑造出杯子形状，然后上颜色。最后，进行高温烧制，这样就做成了杯子。

 Ann：Susan，let's start.
安安：素琴，我们开始吧。

 Susan：First，we will shape the clay into a cup. You must hold the clay carefully because the potter's wheel rotates rapidly. Ann，do you want to give it a shot?
素琴：首先，我们要用陶土塑造出杯子的形状。因为陶工旋盘在快速旋

转，所以你要小心握住陶土。安安，你想试试吗?

 Ann：Susan，it's amazing. I made a cup-like shape.
安：素琴，太神奇了。我做出了杯子形状。

 Susan：Good job Ann. Next，we need to wait for the cup to dry，and then paint it with the color we want.
素琴：做得很好安安。接下来，我们需要等杯子晾干，然后涂上我们喜欢的颜色。

 Ann：I can't wait to paint it.
安安：我已经迫不及待想要涂色了。

词汇

pottery [ˈpɒtəri] n. 陶器
clay [kleɪ] n. 黏土
rotate [rəʊˈteɪt] v. 旋转
rapidly [ˈræpɪdli] adv. 快速地

SING A SONG

对话

 Susan：Halloween is coming. Today，I'm going to teach you a song. *Trick or treat* is the name.
素琴：万圣节快到了。今天我教你们一首儿歌，歌名是《不给糖就捣蛋》。

 Ann：I like Halloween and jack–o'–lantern.
安安：我喜欢万圣节和南瓜灯。

 Susan：Knock knock，trick or treat? Who are you? I'm a witch，I'm a little witch.

Knock knock, trick or treat? Who are you? I'm a monster, I'm a little monster.

Knock knock, trick or treat? Who are you? I'm a pirate. I'm a little pirate.

Knock knock, trick or treat? Happy Halloween! Happy Halloween!

素琴：开门开门，不给糖就捣蛋。你是谁？我是女巫，我是个小女巫。

开门开门，不给糖就捣蛋。你是谁？我是一只怪兽，我是个小怪兽。

开门开门，不给糖就捣蛋。你是谁？我是海盗，我是个小海盗。

开门开门，不给糖就捣蛋。万圣节快乐！万圣节快乐！

Ann：That's a wonderful song. It's very nice.

安安：这歌太棒了，真好听。

Philip：I'm going to dress up as a monster on Halloween and ask grandma for candies.

飞飞：万圣节的时候我要装扮成怪兽，找奶奶要糖。

Ann：I going to dress up as a witch.

安安：我要装扮成女巫。

Susan：OK. Let's sing it together.

素琴：好的。我们一起唱歌吧。

词汇

Halloween ［ˌhæləʊˈiːn］ n. 万圣节

jack - o' - lantern　南瓜灯

monster ［ˈmɒnstə(r)］ n. 怪兽

witch ［wɪtʃ］ n. 女巫

pirate ［ˈpaɪrət］ n. 海盗

ASSEMBLE ROBOT

对话

Philip：Susan, I can't assemble my little robot. Can you help me?

飞飞：素琴，我的小机器人组装不上了。你能帮我吗？

Susan：Don't worry. Let me have a look. Oh honey, you make a mistake with the body part.

素琴：不要着急，让我看一看。哦，亲爱的，身体的部分你组装错了一处。

Philip：Do I need to start over?

飞飞：那我需要重来吗？

Susan：Yes. You'll enjoy the process. It helps to exercise your mind.

素琴：是的。你会喜欢这个过程的。它有助于你锻炼思维。

Philip：Thank you, Susan.

飞飞：谢谢，素琴。

词汇

assemble ［əˈsembl］ vt. 组装

robot ［ˈrəʊbɒt］ n. 机器人

process ［ˈprəʊses］ n. 过程

LEARN SHAPES

对话

Susan：Philip, let's play a game.

素琴：飞飞，我们来玩个游戏。

Philip：What is the game?

飞飞：什么游戏?

Susan：I have a little train here. The train is going to pick up the baby shapes. Each shape has its own seat. When I name the shape, you put it on its seat.

素琴：我这里有一辆小火车。火车要来接这些形状宝宝。每个形状有自己的座位。当我说出这个形状的名字时，你就把它放在它的座位上。

Philip：No problem, Susan.

飞飞：没问题，素琴。

Susan：Let's get started. Number one is circle.

素琴：我们开始吧。第一个是圆形。

Philip：This is the circle.

飞飞：这是圆形。

Susan：Very good. Number two is square.

素琴：非常好，第二个是正方形。

Philip：This is the square.

飞飞：这是正方形。

Susan：Perfect. Number three is triangle.

素琴：完美，第三个是三角形。

Philip：Triangle is seated well.

飞飞：三角形已经坐好了。

Susan：Well done Philip. Number four is rectangle.

素琴：做得很好飞飞，第四个是长方形。

Philip：Rectangle is also seated well.

飞飞：长方形也坐好了。

Susan：Great. The last one is star.

素琴：太棒了。最后一个是星星。

Philip：This is the lovely little star.

飞飞：这是可爱的小星星。

Susan：That's correct. Now all the seats are full, and our little train is leaving.

素琴：没错。现在所有的座位都满了，咱们的小火车要开车了。

词汇

circle ['sɜːkl] n. 圆形

square [skweə(r)] n. 正方形

CLASSIFY THE BUTTONS

对话

Ann：Lots of buttons. They are beautiful.

安安：好多扣子，它们好漂亮。

Susan：Please put those colorful buttons in different bowls according to their sizes, shapes and colors.

素琴：请根据不同的大小、形状、颜色，把这些五颜六色的扣子分别放到不同的碗里。

Ann：These buttons are round and white. I'll put them in the black bowl. There are twelve of them.

安安：这些扣子是圆形白色的，我把它们放在黑色碗里。一共12颗。

Susan：Very good.

素琴：非常好。

59

Ann：Those buttons are dark blue and look like round hats. I'll put them in the gray bowl. There are nine of them. These buttons are lovely pink roses. I'll put them in the orange bowl, and there are ten of them.

安安：这些扣子是深蓝色的，看起来像圆形的帽子。我把它放在灰色的碗里。一共9颗。这些扣子是漂亮的粉色玫瑰花。我把它们放在橙色的碗里，一共10颗。

 Susan：Good job honey. Your observation is very good.

素琴：做得很好亲爱的。你的观察力很强。

词汇

classify ['klæsɪfaɪ] v. 分类
gray [greɪ] n. 灰色
observation [ˌɒbzə'veɪʃn] n. 观察
button ['bʌtn] n. 扣子

CHAPTER FOUR   OUTDOOR ACTIVITIES

RIDE A BIKE （Ⅰ）

对话

Mom：What a nice day today!
妈妈：今天的天气真好！

Ann：I'd like to ride my bike.
安安：我想骑我的自行车。

Mom：It is a tricycle.
妈妈：你的车是三轮车。

Ann：No, it's just a bike with one more wheel.
安安：不，只是自行车多了一个轮子。

Susan：The three wheels help you keep your balance.
素琴：这三个轮子有助于你保持平衡。

Ann：I'd like a bicycle with two wheels. Just like Mom's.
安安：我想要两个轮子的自行车，就像妈妈的一样。

Susan：You haven't ridden a bike.
素琴：你还没有骑过自行车。

Ann：I want to try.
安安：我想试一试。

词汇

ride ［raɪd］ v. 骑
tricycle ［ˈtraɪsɪkl］ n. 三轮车

RIDE A BIKE （Ⅱ）

对话

Dad：I took the stabilizers off the bike. Can you ride a bike without the stabilizers?
爸爸：我刚刚把辅助轮拆了下去。你能不用辅助轮骑自行车吗？

Susan：I think you need some practice.
素琴：我觉得你还需要练习。

Mom：Riding without the stabilizers is not easy.
妈妈：没有辅助轮骑车并不容易。

Ann：I can do it!
安安：我可以的！

Dad：Ann, would you like some help?
爸爸：安安，你想要一些帮助吗？

Ann：Yes, please.
安安：是的。

Dad：go!
爸爸：出发！

Ann：Don't let go.
安安：不要放手。

Dad：Don't worry. I've got you. You are doing really well.

爸爸：别担心，我扶着你呢 。你做得很好。

词汇

stabilizer ['steɪbəlaɪzə(r)] n. （儿童自行车后轮两侧的）稳定轮

RIDE A BIKE（Ⅲ）

对话

Susan：Ann is riding on her own!

素琴：安安正在自己骑自行车!

Ann：Dad, have you let go of the bike?

安安：爸爸，你已经放手了吗?

Dad：Yes, you've been on your own.

爸爸：对，你一直是自己骑。

Ann：Great!

安安：太棒了!

Dad：You're really very good at it!

爸爸：你真的很擅长骑车!

Ann：I don't need the stabilizers anymore!

安安：我再也不用辅助轮了!

Susan：Ann, look out! A slope ahead!

素琴：安安，小心! 前面有一个斜坡!

Ann：Oh, my gosh!

安安：天啊!

Mom：Ann, look ahead.

妈妈：安安，看前面的路。

Dad：When riding, keep in mind to look ahead.

爸爸：骑车时要记得看路。

Ann：I will, Dad.

安安：我会的，爸爸。

词汇

own [əʊn] adj. 自己的
slope [sləʊp] n. 斜坡

GO FOR A SPRING OUTING（Ⅰ）

对话

Susan：We're going to have a spring outing this Saturday.

素琴：我们这个星期六要去春游。

Ann：Great! Where are we going?

安安：太好了! 我们去哪里呢?

Susan：Taifeng Park.

素琴：泰丰公园。

Mom：What should we bring with us?

妈妈：那我们要带些什么?

Susan：We should bring some water, fruit and bread. Because we are going to have picnic there.

素琴：我们要带一些水、水果和面包。因为我们要在那里野餐。

Ann：I'll take my bike with me.

安安：我要带上自行车。

Mom：I'll take my kite.

妈妈：我要带上我的风筝。

Susan：I'll take the tent and mat.

素琴：我要带上帐篷和垫子。

Ann：And the hammock!

安安：还有吊床！

词汇

tent ［tent］ n. 帐篷

mat ［mæt］ n. 垫子

hammock ［'hæmək］ n. 吊床

GO FOR A SPRING OUTING （Ⅱ）

对话

Ann：There are a lot of people out there for a spring outing!

安安：出来春游的人可真多呀！

Susan：We need to find a flat area on the lawn to set up our tent.

素琴：我们需要找一块平坦的草地把帐篷搭起来。

Mom：Over there. Under that big tree.

妈妈：那里，在那棵大树下。

Susan：Good idea!

素琴：好主意！

Ann：Don't forget to secure my hammock.

安安：别忘了把我的吊床系得结实一点。

Susan：Everything is ready. I'd like to enjoy the warm sunshine.

素琴：一切都准备好了。我要享受一下这温暖的阳光。

Mom：There is no wind today. Flying a kite is not easy.

妈妈：今天没有风，不太容易放风筝。

Ann：Let's start with cycling. There is an open space over there.

安安：我们先骑自行车吧。那边有一块空地。

Mom：I want to pick some wild flowers to decorate our tent.

妈妈：我想去采一些野花把我们的帐篷装饰一下。

Ann：I'll go with you.

安安：我和你一起去。

词汇

lawn ［lɔːn］ n. 草坪

wild ［waɪld］ adj. 野生的

decorate ［'dekəreɪt］ vt. 装饰

GO BOATING

对话

Ann：There are many boats on the lake.

安安：湖面上有很多小船。

Mom：I like that yellow boat.

妈妈：我喜欢那个黄色的小船。

Susan：That boat is very beautiful.

素琴：那只小船很漂亮。

Ann：Can we go boating?

安安：我们可以去划船吗？

Susan：There is a ticket office over there.

素琴：售票处在那边。

 Ticket seller：There're two types of boats：the electric powered boat and the pedal boat. Which one do you prefer?
售票员：有两种船。电动船和脚踏船，你们想要哪一种？

 Susan：What are the charges?
素琴：收费是多少？

 Ticket seller：It's 80 *yuan* per hour for an electric boat and 50 *yuan* per hour for a pedal boat.
售票员：电动船 1 小时 80 元，脚踏船 1 小时 50 元。

 Susan：How many people does each boat carry?
素琴：每条船能坐几个人？

 Ticket seller：Up to four people.
售票员：最多能坐 4 个人。

 Susan：We'd like an electric boat.
素琴：我们要电动船吧。

词汇

ticket ［'tɪkɪt］n. 票
electric ［ɪ'lektrɪk］adj. 电动的
pedal ［'pedl］n. 踏板
charge ［tʃɑːdʒ］n. 收费

GO SKATING （Ⅰ）

对话

 Ann：I've never skated before.
安安：我从来没有滑过冰。

 Mom：Skating is fun.
妈妈：滑冰很好玩。

 Ann：Mom, you skate very well.
安安：妈妈，你滑得真好。

 Mom：Can I show you how to skate?
妈妈：我能教你怎么滑冰吗？

 Ann：I always slide and fall. It is impossible. I don't want to skate any longer.
安安：我总是滑倒，太难了。我不想滑冰了。

 Susan：Don't worry. Every beginner learns from falls.
素琴：别担心。每个初学者都是从跌倒中学习的。

 Ann：I still don't know how to skate.
安安：我还是不会滑冰。

 Mom：Skating is sliding and pushing forward with your feet.
妈妈：滑冰是用脚往前推着滑行。

 Ann：Thank you, Mom.
安安：谢谢妈妈。

词汇

skating ［'skeɪtɪŋ］n. 滑冰
beginner ［bɪ'ɡɪnə(r)］n. 初学者

GO SKATING （Ⅱ）

对话

 Ann：I can skate on my own now.
安安：我现在可以自己滑冰了。

 Susan：Well done! Ann is doing really well!

素琴：干得好！安安滑得很好啊！

Mom：Yes, I am a good teacher.
妈妈：是的，我是一个好老师。

Susan：Ann, slow down. You'll bump into someone.
素琴：安安，滑慢一点。不然会撞到别人的。

Ann：How do I stop?
安安：怎么停下来？

Mom：I forgot to show her how to stop.
妈妈：我忘了教她怎么停下来。

Ann：Ah, I can't stop.
安安：啊，我停不下来了。

Susan：Does it hurt?
素琴：摔得疼吗？

Ann：It doesn't matter.
安安：没关系。

Mom：Now I'll show you how to stop.
妈妈：现在我来教你怎么停下来。

Ann：It's very easy.
安安：这个很简单。

Mom：Come on, let's skate.
妈妈：来吧，我们一起滑冰。

词汇

bump [bʌmp] vi. 撞

MAKE A SNOWMAN （Ⅰ）

对话

Mom：It's snowing heavily.
妈妈：雪下得真大。

Ann：Let's make a snowman!
安安：我们来堆雪人吧！

Mom：Let's build the snowman's body.
妈妈：我们来堆雪人的身体。

Ann：I think this body is a little fat.
安安：我觉得这个身体有点胖。

Mom：It doesn't matter. It looks lovely.
妈妈：没关系的，这样显得很可爱。

Ann：I'll make the snowman's head.
安安：我来做雪人的头。

Mom：What a big head!
妈妈：这头可真大呀！

Ann：It looks smart.
安安：这样看起来很聪明。

Mom：Its head is a little crooked.
妈妈：它的头有点歪。

Ann：Maybe it is thinking.
安安：它可能在思考问题。

词汇

crooked ['krʊkɪd] adj. 弯曲的

MAKE A SNOWMAN （Ⅱ）

对话

Mom：I have found two sticks for the snowman's arms.
妈妈：我找了两个树枝来做雪人的胳膊。

Ann：I have found some stones for its eyes and mouth.
安安：我找了几块石头来做它的眼睛

和嘴巴。

Mom：Now the snowman needs a nose.
妈妈：现在雪人还需要一个鼻子。

Ann：Grandma's carrot can be its nose.
安安：奶奶的胡萝卜就可以当鼻子。

Mom：Good idea!
妈妈：好主意!

Ann：Haha, the snowman looks very happy.
安安：哈哈，雪人看起来很开心。

Mom：But maybe it feels cold and needs some warm clothes.
妈妈：但它也许有点冷，需要些暖和衣服。

Ann：Dad's old hat and scarf are just right.
安安：爸爸的旧帽子和围巾正合适。

Mom：Look, this snowman is so handsome!
妈妈：快看呀，这个雪人真帅气!

Susan：This is the best snowman I have ever seen!
素琴：这是我见过的最棒的雪人!

Mom：I think so.
妈妈：我也是这样认为的。

Ann：It's our masterpiece.
安安：它是我们的杰作。

词汇

stick [stɪk] n. 树枝
scarf [skɑːf] n. 围巾
handsome ['hænsəm] adj. 英俊的
masterpiece ['mɑːstəpiːs] n. 杰作

HAVE A SNOWBALL FIGHT

对话

Mom：Ann, let's have a snowball fight.
妈妈：安安，我们来打雪仗吧。

Ann：Great! I'm good at snowball fights.
安安：太好了，我最擅长打雪仗了。

Mom：I think I'll beat you.
妈妈：我想我会打败你的。

Ann：Wait and see.
安安：走着瞧吧。

Mom：First, I must find a fortress.
妈妈：我要先找到一个堡垒。

Ann：I need to make some snowballs.
安安：我要做一些雪球。

Mom：I don't think we need big snowballs. It takes time to make bigger snowballs.
妈妈：我觉得不用太大的雪球，做大雪球费时间。

Ann：But the bigger one is more powerful.
安安：但是大雪球威力更大。

Mom：Do you think my snowball clip works well?
妈妈：你看我的雪球夹子是不是很好用?

Ann：But my hand-made snowball is stronger.
安安：但是我的手工雪球更结实。

Mom：Let's fight.
妈妈：我们开战吧。

词汇

beat ［biːt］vt. 打败（某人）
fortress ［ˈfɔːtrəs］n. 堡垒
clip ［klɪp］n. 夹子
powerful ［ˈpaʊəfl］adj. 强有力的

GO TO THE JUMBLE SALE（Ⅰ）

对话

Mom：I'm going to the school jumble sale today.
妈妈：我今天要去参加学校的义卖活动。

Ann：What is a jumble sale?
安安：什么是义卖活动？

Mom：That is to sell something we don't use anymore at home and donate the money to those who need it.
妈妈：就是把我们家里不再用的东西卖出去，得到的钱捐给需要的人。

Ann：Can I sell my toys?
安安：我可以卖掉我的玩具吗？

Mom：Of course.
妈妈：当然可以。

Ann：What are you going to sell?
安安：你都准备卖些什么？

Mom：My old books and clothes.
妈妈：我的旧书和旧衣服。

Ann：I'm not sure which toy I'd like to sell.

安安：我不确定我要卖掉哪一个玩具。

Mom：You only need to choose one toy.
妈妈：你只需要选择一个玩具就可以了。

Ann：I've decided to sell this toy rabbit because I have a similar one.
安安：我决定把这个玩具兔拿去卖了，因为我还有一只类似的。

Mom：OK，let's go.
妈妈：好的，我们出发吧。

词汇

jumble ［ˈdʒʌmbl］n. 杂乱的一堆东西
sale ［seɪl］n. 销售活动
donate ［dəʊˈneɪt］v. 捐赠
choose ［tʃuːz］v. 选择
decide ［dɪˈsaɪd］v. 决定

GO TO THE JUMBLE SALE（Ⅱ）

对话

Teacher：Hello，everyone. Welcome to this spring's jumble sale. Please take your place.
老师：大家好，欢迎参加今年的春季义卖活动。请大家各就各位。

Mom：Our place is over there.
妈妈：我们的位置在那边。

Susan：It's a good location. It's close to the gate.
素琴：这个位置不错。离大门比较近。

Mom：Yes，everyone will pass by our stall.

妈妈：是的，每个人都会经过我们的摊位。

Ann：It is hot in the sun.

安安：阳光下很炎热。

Mom：There is a sunshade.

妈妈：有一把遮阳伞。

Susan：Great!

素琴：太好了!

Ann：I'm so happy. My rabbit was sold for 2 *yuan*.

安安：我真高兴，我的兔子卖了2元钱。

Mom：We made 16 *yuan* today.

妈妈：我们今天一共赚了16元钱。

Susan：You are a very experienced seller.

素琴：你是一个很有经验的卖家。

Mom：I've been to several jumble sales.

妈妈：我已经参加过好几次义卖了。

词汇

location [ləuˈkeɪʃn] n. 位置
sunshade [ˈsʌnʃeɪd] n. 遮阳伞
experienced [ɪkˈspɪəriənst] adj. 有经验的

PLAY HIDE AND SEEK

对话

Ann：It's my turn to hide.
安安：该轮到我去藏了。

Mom：I'm going to count to ten.

妈妈：我数到十。

Susan：You should count slowly.

素琴：你应该数慢一点。

Mom：Here I come. I will find you.

妈妈：我来了。我一定会找到你的。

Mom：Where could she hide herself?

妈妈：她能藏在哪呢？

Susan：Ann is not behind the big tree.

素琴：安安没在大树后面。

Mom：She's not under the bench either.

妈妈：她也没在椅子下面。

Susan：There is a small shed over there.

素琴：那边有一个小棚子。

Mom：I think she must be there.

妈妈：我想她一定躲在那里边。

Mom：Ann, I found you!

妈妈：安安，我找到你了！

Ann：Haha, it's not easy to find me here!

安安：哈哈，在这里找到我并不容易吧！

词汇

seek [si:k] v. 寻找

JUMP ROPE

对话

Ann：Let's jump rope in the public square.

68

安安：我们到广场去跳绳吧。

 Susan：How many jumps can you make?

素琴：你能跳多少个？

 Ann：I'm not sure, but it doesn't look too difficult.

安安：我不确定，但这看起来并不太难。

 Susan：I'll count for you. One, two, three, four, five…

素琴：我来给你数数 1、2、3、4、5……

 Ann：I think I need to practice.

安安：我想我需要练习。

 Susan：It would be easier to jump over if your rope is shorter.

素琴：如果你的绳子再短一点会更容易跳。

 Ann：Yes, it's much better.

安安：是的，这样好多了。

 Susan：You've done 30 jumps.

素琴：你已经跳了 30 下了。

 Ann：I can jump more.

安安：我能跳得更多。

 Susan：As long as you practice more, you will jump more.

素琴：只要多多练习就会跳得更多。

词汇

rope［rəʊp］n. 绳子

square［skweə(r)］n. 广场

PICK FRUIT

对话

 Susan：We are going to pick strawberries in the orchard today.

素琴：我们今天要去果园采摘草莓。

 Mom：Do we take any containers with us?

妈妈：我们要带一些容器吗？

 Susan：Each of us takes a small basket. We also need to wear sports clothes and comfortable shoes.

素琴：我们每个人带一个小篮子。我们还要穿运动衣和舒服的鞋。

 Ann：It's too hot in the strawberry shed.

安安：草莓棚里太热了。

 Susan：You can take off your jacket.

素琴：你可以把外套脱掉。

 Mom：These strawberries must be very sweet.

妈妈：这些草莓一定很甜。

 Ann：Yes, they are big and red.

安安：对，它们又大又红。

 Susan：Let's pick them gently. Don't bruise the strawberries.

素琴：我们要轻轻摘，别把草莓碰坏了。

 Ann：Can I have a strawberry?

安安：我可以吃一个草莓吗？

 Susan：We must wash it before you eat it.

69

素琴：吃之前一定要洗一洗。

Ann：I want to share these strawberries with my good friends.
安安：我想把这些草莓分给我的好朋友们。

Susan：Your friends will be very happy.
素琴：你的朋友们一定会很开心。

词汇

orchard [ˈɔːtʃəd] n. 果园

RIDE THE CABLE CAR

对话

Mom：I am too tired to go any further.
妈妈：我太累了，走不动了。

Ann：Me too. Let's take a cable car.
安安：我也是。我们坐缆车吧。

Mom：There are so many people in line.
妈妈：排队的人可真多。

Susan：Be patient. It's better to wait than to walk.
素琴：耐心点。等着总比走着好。

Ann：The cable car is like a cabin!
安安：缆车像一个小屋！

Susan：The view of the scenery from the cable car is really beautiful.
素琴：在缆车上看景色真的很美呀。

Ann：But it is too high. I am a little scared.
安安：可是缆车实在是太高了，我有

点害怕。

Mom：Don't look down. Look ahead in the distance.
妈妈：别看下边，向远方看。

Ann：It seems like I can touch the clouds.
安安：我好像能碰到云。

Susan：Wait a minute. Let's take a picture.
素琴：等一下，我们来拍一张照片。

Ann：Yes, in memory of my first cable car ride.
安安：对，来纪念我第一次坐缆车。

词汇

cable [ˈkeɪbl] n. 缆绳
scenery [ˈsiːnəri] n. 景色
memory [ˈmeməri] n. 回忆

WATCH LANTERNS

对话

Mom：The lanterns of this year are better than last year.
妈妈：今年的花灯比去年的好看。

Susan：This year, many people have come to watch the lanterns.
素琴：今年来看花灯的人很多。

Ann：I like that red lantern.
安安：我喜欢那个红色的灯笼。

Susan：I think the blue one is also very beautiful.
素琴：我觉得那个蓝色的花灯也很

漂亮。

Mom：I like that rainbow lantern.
妈妈：我喜欢那个彩虹灯笼。

Ann：There is a snake over there.
安安：那边有一条蛇。

Mom：And a dragon.
妈妈：还有一条龙。

Susan：These are the lanterns of the Chinese zodiac.
素琴：这些是生肖灯笼。

Ann：This is my zodiac. It's a rabbit.
安安：这是我的生肖，它是一只兔子。

Mom：Mine is a rat.
妈妈：我的是一只老鼠。

Susan：They are so lovely！
素琴：它们都好可爱呀！

Mom：Take a look at the moon. It's like a lantern，too.
妈妈：快看天上的月亮。它也像一个灯笼。

词汇

dragon ['drægən] n. 龙
Chinese zodiac 生肖

TAKE PART IN SPORTS EVENTS

对话

Ann：Today is the school sports day.
安安：今天学校开运动会。

Susan：How many sports events do you have today?
素琴：你们都有哪些比赛项目？

Ann：High jump，long jump，50m race and relay race.
安安：跳高、跳远、50 米跑和接力比赛。

Mom：Are you going to take part in any of the events?
妈妈：你会参加哪个项目？

Ann：I'm going to take part in the 50m race.
安安：我要参加 50 米跑。

Susan：You are cut out for this event. You run very fast.
素琴：这个项目太适合你了。你跑得很快。

Mom：I'm going to cheer you on.
妈妈：我要去给你加油。

Ann：I will fight for the first place.
安安：我要力争得到第一名。

Susan：Ann is in the lead.
素琴：安安一路领先。

Mom：Come on！Come on！
妈妈：加油！加油！

Susan：Ann wins the race.
素琴：安安赢得了比赛。

词汇

race [reɪs] n. 赛跑
lead [liːd] n. 领先地位

GO FOR A WALK

对话

Ann：It's boring.
安安：太无聊了。

Susan：Do you want to go for a walk in the park?
素琴：你想不想到公园里去走走?

Ann：A walk in the park?
安安：到公园里走走?

Susan：It's neither cold nor hot today. The peach blossoms in the park are blooming. I'm going for a walk.
素琴：今天不冷也不热，公园的桃花也开了，我要去散散步。

Ann：Are there peach blossoms in the park? I'm going to pick up some petals to make bookmarkers.
安安：公园里有桃花? 我要去捡一些花瓣做成书签。

Susan：Let's go.
素琴：我们出发吧。

Ann：The air is fresh here.
安安：这里的空气真新鲜。

Susan：The sun is shining brightly.
素琴：阳光真明媚。

Ann：I can smell the scent of flowers.
安安：我闻到了花香。

Susan：There is a peach blossom grove over there.
素琴：那边有一片桃花林。

Ann：Many people have come to watch the peach blossoms.
安安：很多人都来看桃花。

Susan：There are many colors of the peach blossoms.
素琴：有很多种颜色的桃花。

Ann：White, pink and red.
安安：有白的、粉的和红的。

Susan：Taking a walk here gives me better mood.
素琴：在这里散步我心情真好。

词汇

blossom ['blɒsəm] n. 花朵
fresh [freʃ] adj. 新鲜的

GO TO THE ZOO（Ⅰ）

对话

Ann：I want to go to the zoo.
安安：我想去动物园。

Philip：I want to go to the zoo too.
飞飞：我也想去动物园。

Ann：Mommy, could we go to the zoo?
安安：妈妈，我们能去动物园吗?

Philip：Mommy, I want to see the tigers.
飞飞：妈妈，我想去看老虎。

Mom：Okay, let us go to the zoo.
妈妈：好的，我们去动物园吧。

Ann：Hooray! We're going to the zoo!
安安：好哇! 我们要去动物园啦!

词汇

hooray ［huˈreɪ］int.（表示快乐或赞同）好极了

GO TO THE ZOO（Ⅱ）

对话

Philip：Is the zoo far away？
飞飞：动物园远吗？

Mom：The zoo is not far away from our home．It takes 10 minutes by car．
妈妈：动物园离我们家不远，开车去需要 10 分钟。

Ann：I would like to take a bus, a double-decker bus！
安安：我想坐公交车，双层巴士！

Mom：Daddy will drop us off at the zoo, but we can take a double-decker bus home．Is that OK？
妈妈：爸爸开车送我们去动物园，但是我们可以乘双层巴士回家，好吗？

Ann：Okay, but why doesn't Daddy go to the zoo with us？
安安：好吧，但是爸爸为什么不和我们一起进动物园呢？

Mom：Daddy is on duty today．Susan will go with us．
妈妈：爸爸今天值班。素琴和我们一起去。

Susan：Children, we'll have a ball.
素琴：孩子们，我们会玩得很开心的！

词汇

double-decker bus　双层巴士
on duty　值班
have a ball　玩儿得开心，过得愉快

GO TO THE ZOO（Ⅲ）

对话

Susan：Look, that is the petting zoo area．
素琴：看，那是宠物区。

Mom：Let's feed the little animals．
妈妈：我们喂小动物吧。

Ann：Little rabbit, here is the carrot for you．
安安：小兔子，这是给你的胡萝卜。

Philip：Calf, here is the cabbage for you．
飞飞：小牛，这是给你的圆白菜。

Ann：Foal, here is the Chinese cabbage for you．
安安：小马驹，这是给你的大白菜。

Susan：We also have some popcorn for the goats．
素琴：我们还有爆米花，可以喂小山羊。

Ann：Isn't that for us？
安安：那不是给我们的吗？

Susan：This is sugar－free popcorn especially for little animals．Would you like to have a taste？
素琴：这是专给小动物们的无糖爆米

73

花，你要尝一尝吗？

Ann：Hmm, the sugar - free popcorn tastes good.
安安：嗯，没有糖的爆米花好吃。

Mom：Honey, save some for the goats!
妈妈：宝贝，给山羊留一些！

词汇

calf ［kɑːf］ n. 小牛
foal ［fəʊl］ n. 小马驹
cabbage ［ˈkæbɪdʒ］ n. 圆白菜
Chinese cabbage 大白菜
popcorn ［ˈpɒpkɔːn］ n. 爆米花

GO TO THE ZOO （Ⅳ）

对话

Susan：This is the departure station for the sightseeing shuttle buses that take us to the beast area.
素琴：这是去猛兽区的游览车发车站。

Mom：Let's get in line.
妈妈：我们来排队吧。

Ann：What animals live in the beast area?
安安：什么动物生活在猛兽区？

Susan：Tigers, lions, bears, wolves, leopards and the like.
素琴：老虎、狮子、熊、狼、豹子一类的动物。

Philip：Tiger, tiger, I will see you soon!
飞飞：老虎，老虎，我很快就能看到

你了！

Susan：Look over there, there are two tigers with heavy black stripes on their orange coats.
素琴：看那边，有两只老虎，它们的橙色皮毛上有很深的黑色条纹。

Ann：Are tigers all in orange and black?
安安：老虎都是橙黑相间的吗？

Mom：White tigers have a coat that is white with black stripes on it. Some of the rarer white tigers are completely white in color.
妈妈：白虎的皮毛是白色带黑条纹，有些罕见的白虎是纯白色的。

Susan：There are two white tigers in the beast area that are completely white.
素琴：猛兽区有两只纯白的白虎。

Ann：That is so cool!
安安：好酷啊！

词汇

sightseeing shuttle bus 游览车
strip ［strɪp］ n. 条纹

GO TO THE ZOO （Ⅴ）

对话

Mom：There are a lot of parrots.
妈妈：这有很多鹦鹉。

Ann：Can parrots talk?
安安：鹦鹉会说话吗？

Mom：Parrots are very intelligent. They have the ability to talk.

妈妈：鹦鹉很聪明，它们能说话。

Ann：Hello，parrot，can you say hello? Mom，it doesn't talk.

安安：你好，鹦鹉，你能打个招呼吗? 妈妈，它不说话。

Mom：Most parrots learn to talk when they are either kept alone with humans or with other parrots who talk.

妈妈：大多数鹦鹉是在与人类或其他会说话的鹦鹉独处时学习说话的。

Ann：How about feeding it while teaching it the word—eat?

安安：在喂它的时候教它"吃"这个词怎么样?

Mom：It is a good idea. Let's buy some bird feed.

妈妈：这是个好主意。我们去买些鸟饲料。

Ann：I've got a piece of chocolate. He might enjoy it.

安安：我有一块巧克力，也许它喜欢吃。

Mom：No，honey，chocolates contain something toxic to birds.

妈妈：不可以，亲爱的，巧克力中含有对鸟类有毒的物质。

Ann：How about some chips?

安安：来点薯片怎么样?

Mom：Chips are high-salt food，which can be harmful to them.

妈妈：薯片是高盐食物，对它们可能有害。

Ann：I see.

安安：我明白了。

词汇

intelligent［ɪnˈtelɪdʒənt］adj. 聪明的

feed［fiːd］n. 饲料

toxic［ˈtɒksɪk］adj. 有毒的

GO PICNIC（Ⅰ）

对话

Mom：What a lovely weather today!

妈妈：今天天气真好!

Susan：It is not half sunny.

素琴：天气非常晴朗。

Mom：Let's go picnic.

妈妈：我们去野餐吧。

Susan：Where are we going to have the picnic?

素琴：我们去哪野餐呢?

Mom：Let's go to the park.

妈妈：我们去公园吧。

Susan：We have sandwiches，bananas，cakes and chips. Who would like a slice of cake?

素琴：我们有三明治、香蕉、蛋糕和薯条。谁想要块蛋糕?

Philip：I'd like one，please.

飞飞：我想要一块。

Ann：I'd like a sandwich and a banana.

安安：我要三明治和香蕉。

Susan：You like bananas very much, don't you?

素琴：你很喜欢吃香蕉，是不是？

 Ann：Not half.

安安：非常。

词汇

chips［tʃɪps］n. 炸薯条

GO PICNIC（Ⅱ）

对话

 Mom：Look, there is a campsite in the meadow.

妈妈：看，草地那有一处露营地。

 Dad：Phil, would you give me a hand to set up the tent?

爸爸：飞飞，帮我搭帐篷好吗？

Philip：OK.

飞飞：好。

 Dad：We need a very flat site to lay out all the parts of the tent on the tarp. First, connect the tent poles.

爸爸：我们需要一个非常平坦的地方，把帐篷的所有零件放在防水布上。首先，把帐篷杆连接上。

 Philip：Like this?

飞飞：像这样吗？

 Dad：Yes, well done, Phil.

爸爸：对的，飞飞做得很好。

Philip：Where do these poles go?

飞飞：这些杆插哪？

 Dad：Insert the tips of each pole into these eyelets.

爸爸：杆头插到这些小孔里。

 Philip：Daddy, let me try.

飞飞：爸爸，让我试一下。

 Dad：Now, let's raise the tent.

爸爸：现在，我们举起帐篷。

 Philip：We set the tent!

飞飞：我们搭好帐篷啦！

 Dad：Not yet, Phil. One more step. Let's fix the tent to the ground.

爸爸：还没有，飞飞。还有一个步骤，我们把帐篷固定到地上吧。

 Philip：How do we fix the tent?

飞飞：怎么固定帐篷？

 Dad：Push the stake through and into the ground to secure the tent.

爸爸：把固定桩扎到地上固定帐篷。

词汇

campsite［ˈkæmpsaɪt］n. 野营地

meadow［ˈmedəʊ］n. 草地

tarp［tɑːp］n. 防水布

pole［pəʊl］n. 杆

insert［ɪnˈsɜːt］v. 插入

eyelets［ˈaɪlət］n. 孔眼

stake［steɪk］n. 桩

secure［sɪˈkjʊə(r)］v. 使固定

GO PICNIC（Ⅲ）

对话

 Susan：It's windy, let's fly a kite!

素琴：起风了，我们放风筝吧。

Mom：Let's look for an open space that is free of trees and power lines.

妈妈：我们找一个没有树和电线的空地。

 Susan：Ann，hold the kite in your hands and throw it up into the air to catch a wind.

素琴：安安，双手拿着风筝，把它向上扔到空中让风托起。

 Ann：Oh no，this kite isn't going to fly!

安安：哦，不，这个风筝飞不起来!

 Susan：Honey，try to hold up the kite by the bridle. Phil，would you hold the spool in your hand and run with the kite behind you as soon as your sister toss it into the wind?

素琴：宝贝，试试在提线这里举起风筝。飞飞，你来拿着线轴，当姐姐抛出风筝后，带着风筝向前跑。

 Philip：I can run very fast!

飞飞：我能跑得非常快!

 Susan：The wind lifts it! Phil，let out the string. The more string you let out the higher your kite will fly.

素琴：风把风筝托起来了! 飞飞放线。你放出的线越多，风筝就会飞得越高。

词汇

open space　空地

bridle［ˈbraɪdl］n. 提线

spool［spuːl］n. 线轴

toss［tɒs］v. 抛

string［strɪŋ］n. 线

GO PICNIC （Ⅳ）

对话

 Susan：Ann，Phil，do you want to play tag?

素琴：安安，飞飞，想玩儿抓人吗?

 Ann：Who is the tagger?

安安：谁当抓人的人?

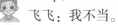 Philip：I am not "it".

飞飞：我不当。

 Susan：Well，let's decide "it" by playing rock，paper and scissors.

素琴：那我们用剪刀石头布决定吧。

 Mom：I'm "it". I'll count to ten to give you time to run away. 1，2，3，4，5，6，7，8，9，10. Ready or not? Here I come!

妈妈：我是来抓人的。我给你们10秒钟的时间先跑。1，2，3，4，5，6，7，8，9，10。准备好了吗? 我来了。

 Susan：Ann，Phil，run away. Whoever being tagged will become "it".

素琴：安安，飞飞，跑远点。被抓到就会成为抓人的人。

 Ann：Mommy，you can't get me.

安安：妈妈你抓不到我。

 Philip：Mommy，come and catch me!

飞飞：妈妈来抓我吧!

 Mom：I'm about to catch you! You're tagged.

77

妈妈：我快要抓到你了！你被抓了！

Philip：Now, it's my turn to catch you!

飞飞：现在轮到我抓你们啦！

Susan：Phil, you are really fast. I am out of breath. I'm exhausted!

素琴：飞飞，你跑得真快。我上不来气，没力气了！

Philip：You are slower than me. You're tagged.

飞飞：你比我跑得慢。你被抓了。

词汇

play tag 玩抓人游戏

tagger [ˈtægə(r)] n. 抓人的人

exhausted [ɪgˈzɔːstɪd] adj. 筋疲力尽的

GO PICNIC（Ⅴ）

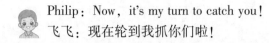

对话

Susan：The weather is changing. It was cloudy when we were playing tag, and it is overcast now.

素琴：变天啦。刚才我们玩儿抓人的时候是多云，现在是阴云密布。

Mom：Kids, we'd better go home or we'll be caught in the rain.

妈妈：孩子们，我们最好回家，否则会淋雨。

Susan：The wind is stronger and it's drizzling now.

素琴：风更大了，而且下毛毛雨了。

Ann：Woops, a gust of wind just blew my hat away!

安安：糟糕，刚才一阵大风把我的帽子吹跑了！

Susan：It's there, I'll get it.

素琴：它在那里，我去拿吧。

Mom：Honey, there is a flash of lightning. We'd better leave before the rain pours down.

妈妈：宝贝儿，打闪电了。我们最好在下大雨前离开。

Ann：Can I play a little longer?

安安：我能再玩儿会吗?

Mom：The rain is coming down. You may get wet in the rain and catch a cold. Besides, it is not safe to stay outside in thunderstorm days.

妈妈：雨下起来了。你可能会淋雨感冒的，而且雷雨天气在户外不安全。

Susan：Let's go back home. When the rain gets lighter, you can put on your raincoat and rain boots to play outside.

素琴：我们先回家吧，等雨小些，你可以穿上雨衣和雨鞋在外面玩儿。

Ann：All right, I want to jump in muddy puddles. I want to find a big puddle.

安安：好的，我想玩儿跳泥坑，我要找个大坑。

Susan：Fine, we'll jump in muddy puddles together!

素琴：好，我们一起玩儿跳泥坑！

词汇

overcast [ˌəʊvəˈkɑːst] a. 阴天的

drizzle [ˈdrɪzl] vi. 下毛毛雨

lightning [ˈlaɪtnɪŋ] n. 闪电

pour [pɔː(r)] v. （雨）倾盆而下

GO TO THE ROLE PLAY THEME PARK（Ⅰ）

对话

Docent：Welcome to our role play theme park！This area shows you how firefighters work. Here are the different personal protective equipment and tools used by firefighters.

讲解员：欢迎来到我们的职业体验馆。这个区域介绍的是消防员如何工作。这些是消防员使用的个人防护设备和不同的工具。

Ann：So, a firefighter must put on an orange jacket and trousers, as well as a helmet and face mask.

安安：消防员需要穿上橘色的外套和裤子，戴上头盔和面罩。

Docent：Yes. Do you know what makes this orange jacket different from yours?

讲解员：是的。你知道这个橙色外套和你的橙色外套有什么区别吗？

Ann：Is it much bigger?

安安：更大？

Docent：It is flame-resistant and insu-lated, keeping firefighters safe from high temperatures and water.

讲解员：它具有阻燃性和绝缘性，可帮助消防员抵抗高温和水。

Ann：What is that?

安安：那是什么？

Docent：Oh, that is the self-contained breathing apparatus（SCBA）, which allows a firefighter to breathe inside a smoke-filled building. Do you know why flashlights and axes are used?

讲解员：哦，那是自给式呼吸器（SCBA），它可使消防员在充满烟雾的建筑物内呼吸。你们知道为什么要使用手电筒和斧子吗？

Ann：Firefighters can see in dark buildings with flashlights and break through doors with axes.

安安：手电筒能让消防员在黑暗的建筑里看得见，斧子用来破门。

Docent：Perfect, firefighters are trained to rescue people from a variety of circumstances, and they need these tools.

讲解员：非常棒，消防员受过训练，可以从各种状况下救助人们，他们需要这些工具。

Docent：Kids, let's put on firefighter uniforms and play the role of firefighters now.

讲解员：孩子们，现在让我们穿上消防员的制服，体验消防员的角色吧。

词汇

Role Play Theme Park　职业体验馆
docent［ˈdəʊsnt］n. 讲解员
firefighter［ˈfaɪəfaɪtə(r)］n. 消防员
personal protective equipment　个人防护装备
helmet［ˈhelmɪt］n. 头盔
flame-resistant　耐火的
insulated［ˈɪnsjuleɪtɪd］adj. 绝缘的
self-contained breathing apparatus　自给式呼

吸器

breathe ［briːð］ v. 呼吸

circumstance ［ˈsɜːkəmstəns］ n. 状况

GO TO THE ROLE PLAY THEME PARK（Ⅱ）

对话

Docent：Welcome to the doctor's area. Do you know what is this instrument?

讲解员：欢迎来到医生展区。你们知道这是什么器械吗？

Ann：It's a stethoscope.

安安：听诊器。

Docent：Good. As you can see, a stethoscope consists of a bell-shaped device, a length of rubber tubing, and a headset with two earpieces. Who can show me where I place the 'bell'?

讲解员：很好。如你所见，听诊器由一个钟形装置、一段橡胶管和一个带有两个听筒的耳机组成。谁可以告诉我，这个"钟"应该放在哪里？

Ann：My doctor placed it on my chest and back, asking me to take a deep breath.

安安：我的医生把它放在我的胸部和背部，还让我深呼吸。

Docent：You are observant, aren't you? As you take deep breaths, sounds from your chest cavity travel through the rubber tube and headset, reaching the doctor's ears through these two earpieces. Who would like to listen to my heartbeats?

讲解员：你很善于观察，对吗？深呼吸时，来自胸腔的声音通过橡胶管和耳机传播，并通过两个听筒到达医生的耳朵。谁想听听我的心跳？

Ann：May I give a shot? I can hear the 'lub-dub, lub-dub, lub-dub' sounds.

安安：我可以尝试一下吗？我可以听到"扑通，扑通，扑通"的声音。

Docent：It's my heart beating. You can also hear heartbeats of this manikin through the stethoscope.

讲解员：这是我的心跳。您还可以通过听诊器听到这个模拟人的心跳。

Ann：Is it alive?

安安：它是活的吗？

Docent：No, it's a model of human body. But it allows us to hear heartbeats, take temperature and pulse, and check pupil reflex.

讲解员：不，这是人体模型。但它能让我们听到心跳，测量体温和脉搏，检查瞳孔反射。

词汇

instrument ［ˈɪnstrəmənt］ n. 器械

stethoscope ［ˈsteθəskəʊp］ n. 听诊器

length ［leŋθ］ n. 长度

rubber ［ˈrʌbə(r)］ n. 橡胶

tubing ［ˈtjuːbɪŋ］ n. 管

headset ［ˈhedset］ n. 耳机

earpiece ［ˈɪəpiːs］ n. 听筒

observant ［əbˈzɜːvənt］ adj. 善于观察的

heartbeat ［ˈhɑːtbiːt］ n. 心跳

lub-dub （心跳）扑通声

pulse ［pʌls］ n. 脉搏

pupil ［ˈpjuːpl］ n. 瞳孔

reflex ［ˈriːfleks］ n. 反射动作

GO TO THE ROLE PLAY THEME PARK（Ⅲ）

对话

 Docent：Welcome to the cook's area. A cook is a person who prepares and cooks food. What is your favorite food?
讲解员：欢迎来到厨师区。厨师是准备和烹饪食物的人。你最喜欢什么食物？

 Ann：I like sweet potatoes.
安安：我喜欢红薯。

 Docent：What's your favorite dish?
讲解员：你最喜欢的一道菜是什么？

 Ann：I like pancakes very much. My mom always makes pancakes for breakfast. Sometimes, she asks me to help.
安安：我非常喜欢蔬菜煎饼。我妈妈早餐经常做煎饼。有时候，她让我帮忙。

 Docent：I bet you are an excellent cook！Would you like to make a pancake for your mom today? You can use the kitchen wares and ingredients here.
讲解员：我敢说，你是一名优秀的厨师！你今天想给妈妈做个煎饼吗？你可以使用这里的厨房用品和原材料。

 Ann：Mom, I'll make you a pancake. Would you please give me a hand?
安安：妈妈，我给你做个煎饼。你能

帮我一下吗？

 Mom：Thank you, honey. I'd love to. We need eggs, flour and grated vegetables.
妈妈：谢谢你，亲爱的，我很乐意帮忙。我们需要鸡蛋、面粉和磨碎的蔬菜。

 Ann：Mom, I'll put them all together in this large bowl. Would you heat the oil?
安安：妈妈，我会把它们混合在这个大碗里。你能把油加热吗？

 Mom：Sure.
妈妈：当然可以。

 Ann：It smells so good.
安安：闻起来真香。

词汇

cook ［kʊk］ n. 厨师
kitchen wares   n. 厨房用品
ingredient ［ɪnˈɡriːdiənt］ n.（烹调的）原料
grate ［ˈɡreɪt］ vt. 磨碎

GO TO THE ROLE PLAY THEME PARK（Ⅳ）

对话

 Docent：Welcome to the grocery cashier's area. A grocery cashier totals up customers' purchases, counting and handling money.
讲解员：欢迎来到食品杂货店收银员区。收银员汇总顾客的购物金额，清点并经手钱款。

Ann：Is this a computer?
安安：这是一台电脑吗？

Docent：This is a cash register. This is a bar-code scanner.
讲解员：这是收银机。这是条形码扫描仪。

Ann：It's the same scanner as the one at 7-Eleven.
安安：和 7 – 11 的扫描仪是一样的。

Docent：Do you have any idea where a cashier scans with a scanner?
讲解员：你知道收银员用扫描仪扫描哪里吗？

Ann：At the label of the bar-code.
安安：扫描条形码标签。

Docent：Exactly. Would you like to give a shot?
讲解员：非常正确。你想试试吗？

Ann：Yes. Mom, would you pretend to be a customer?
安安：想试试。妈妈，你可以假装是顾客吗？

Mom：OK, these are the things I want to buy. How much is it?
妈妈：好的，这些是我买的东西。多少钱？

Ann：It's 60 *yuan*.
安安：60 元。

Mom：Can you make change for 100 *yuan*?
妈妈：你能找开 100 元吗？

Ann：Yes. 100 minus 60 equals 40. Here is your 40 *yuan* and receipt. Thanks for coming.

安安：可以。100 减 60 等于 40. 这是你的 40 元钱和收据。谢谢你的光临。

词汇

grocery ［'grəʊsəri］ n. 食品杂货店

cashier ［kæ'ʃɪə(r)］ n. 收银员

customer ［'kʌstəmə(r)］ n. 顾客

purchase ［'pɜːtʃəs］ n. 购买的东西

change ［tʃeɪndʒ］ n. 零钱

bar-code 条形码

scanner ［'skænə(r)］ n. 扫描器

cash register 收银机

minus ［'maɪnəs］ prep. 减去

equal ［'iːkwəl］ v. 等于

receipt ［rɪ'siːt］ n. 收据

GO TO THE ROLE PLAY THEME PARK（Ⅴ）

对话

Docent：Welcome to the teacher's area. A teacher teaches students and helps them learn by themselves.
讲解员：欢迎来到教师区。教师教学生，也帮助学生自学。

Ann：I like my Chinese teacher very much. She is very kind and patient.
安安：我非常喜欢我的语文老师。她人很好，而且有耐心。

Docent：I'm glad to hear that you've had a good time at school. How does your Chinese teacher teach in class?
讲解员：我很高兴你喜欢学校生活。你的语文老师在课堂上怎样讲课？

Ann：She uses a projector to display Chinese characters on a screen, then writes them on the blackboard with chalk. She always names some students to write on the blackboard as well.

安安：她用投影仪在屏幕上打出汉字，然后用粉笔把这些汉字写在黑板上。她也会叫一些学生在黑板上写字。

Docent：Have you been asked to write on the blackboard?

讲解员：你有被叫去在黑板上写字吗？

Ann：Yes, and as a reward, I got a sticker.

安安：是的，我还得到了一张贴纸作为奖励。

Docent：Good for you!

讲解员：你真棒！

词汇

character［ˈkærəktə(r)］n. 文字

chalk［tʃɔːk］n. 粉笔

sticker［ˈstɪkə(r)］n. 贴纸

reward［rɪˈwɔːd］n. 奖励

GO TO THE MARINE PARK（Ⅰ）

对话

Ann：Look, penguins!

安安：看，企鹅！

Mom：Penguins are birds that do not fly.

妈妈：企鹅是不会飞的鸟。

Ann：Do they have feathers?

安安：它们有羽毛吗？

Mom：Yes, they have a thick layer of feathers that keep them warm in the water.

妈妈：有的，它们有一层厚厚的羽毛，使它们在水中保持温暖。

Ann：Look, Mommy, a little penguin is waddling on his feet.

安安：看，妈妈，一只小企鹅摇摇晃晃地走起来了。

Mom：This one is sliding on his belly.

妈妈：这只正在用肚皮滑行。

Ann：They are so cute. What do penguins eat?

安安：它们真可爱。企鹅吃什么？

Mom：They eat fish.

妈妈：吃鱼。

Ann：How could they catch the fish?

安安：它们怎么抓鱼的呢？

Mom：They catch the fish with their beaks and then swallow it.

妈妈：它们用喙抓住鱼，然后把鱼吞下去。

Ann：Wow, that's amazing.

安安：哇，太棒了。

词汇

layer［ˈleɪə(r)］n. 层

waddle［ˈwɒdl］vi.（像鸭子一样）摇摇摆摆地走

beak［biːk］n. 鸟喙

83

GO TO THE MARINE PARK（Ⅱ）

对话

Ann：Wow！How big polar bears are！
安安：北极熊好大啊！

Dad：Yes，they are.
爸爸：是的。

Ann：What do polar bears eat？
安安：北极熊吃什么呢？

Dad：Polar bears like to eat seals very much.
爸爸：北极熊非常喜欢吃海豹。

Ann：Dad，why can polar bears live in such cold places as the Arctic？
安安：爸爸，为什么北极熊能在北极那样寒冷的地方生活呢？

Dad：Polar bears have fat layers that keep them warm.
爸爸：北极熊有脂肪层，可以让它们保持体温。

Ann：My teacher said that polar bears are listed as a threatened species.
安安：老师说，北极熊被列为濒危物种了。

Dad：Yes，global warming is the most serious threat to polar bears.
爸爸：是的，全球气候变暖是北极熊面临的最大威胁。

Ann：What should we do to help them？
安安：我们该怎么帮助它们呢？

Dad：Let's begin to protect the environment by saving energy and reducing carbon dioxide emissions. How about we take a bus home today？
爸爸：让我们通过节约能源，减少二氧化碳排放保护环境吧。今天咱们坐公交车回家怎么样？

Ann：OK.
安安：好的。

词汇

the Arctic　北极地区
threatened［ˈθretnd］adj. 受到威胁的
species［ˈspiːʃiːz］n. 物种
carbon dioxide　二氧化碳
energy［ˈenədʒi］n. 能源
emission［iˈmiʃn］n. 排放

GO TO THE MARINE PARK（Ⅲ）

对话

Dad：Do you know that jellyfish are not fish？
爸爸：你知道水母不是鱼吗？

Ann：What are they？
安安：它们是什么？

Dad：They are soft round sea animals.
爸爸：它们是柔软的圆形海洋动物。

Ann：What do jellyfish eat？
安安：水母吃什么？

Dad：They are likely to eat fish and other jellyfish.
爸爸：它们有可能会吃鱼和其他

水母。

Ann：Jellyfish looks so harmless.
安安：水母看起来很无害。

Dad：While they may look harmless, most jellyfish are stinging.
爸爸：虽然它们看起来无害，但大多数水母都可以蛰人。

Ann：Where is the mouth of the jellyfish?
安安：水母的嘴在哪里？

Dad：Look at the jelly-like body, and you will notice a small hole at the bottom. That is the mouth of the jellyfish.
爸爸：看看这个果冻一样的身体，你会发现它的底部有一个小洞。那是水母的嘴。

Ann：That is weird.
安安：好奇怪。

词汇

harmless [ˈhɑːmləs] adj. 无害的
stinging [ˈstɪŋɪŋ] adj. 蛰人的

GO TO THE MARINE PARK（Ⅳ）

对话

Ann：Take a look at the little white foxes, they are so cute.
安安：看这个小白狐狸，真可爱。

Dad：These are the arctic foxes. They wear a white coat during winter and a brown coat in the summer.
爸爸：它们是北极狐。它们冬天有一件白色的外套，夏天有一件棕色的外套。

Ann：Couldn't they be spotted if they have brown coats in the summer?
安安：如果夏天穿棕色外套，它们不是会被发现吗？

Dad：In the summer, the Arctic has a variety of colours. The arctic foxes' brown coats blend with the summer background.
爸爸：夏天的北极有不同的颜色。北极狐的棕色皮毛与夏天的背景能够融为一体。

Ann：They are so smart.
安安：它们太聪明了。

Dad：They also have small noses, eyes, and ears to keep the body heat from escaping.
爸爸：它们的鼻子、眼睛和耳朵也很小，以防止身体热量逸出。

Ann：What do arctic foxes eat?
安安：北极狐吃什么？

Dad：Birds, bird eggs and berries.
爸爸：鸟、鸟蛋和浆果。

词汇

arctic [ˈɑːktɪk] adj. 北极的
blend [blend] v. （颜色）融合
escape [ɪˈskeɪp] vi. （气体、液体等）漏出

CHAPTER FIVE HEALTH CARE

HAVE FEVER

对话

Mom：Good morning!

妈妈：早上好!

Philip：Mom, I am not feeling very well!

飞飞：妈妈，我觉得不太舒服。

Mom：What's the matter? Come over here. Let me have a look!

妈妈：怎么了？过来让我看看!

Philip：I have a headache.

飞飞：我头疼。

Mom：Let me take your temperature.

妈妈：我给你测一下体温吧。

Philip：Do I have a fever?

飞飞：我发烧了吗？

Mom：Yes, your temperature is 37.8 degrees.

妈妈：是的，你的体温是 37.8 度。

Philip：Mom, do I need to take some medicine?

飞飞：妈妈，我要吃药吗？

Mom：I'm going to call Dr. Wang and ask for his advice.

妈妈：我要给王医生打个电话，听听他的建议。

Philip：Do I have to go to kindergarten today?

飞飞：我今天还去幼儿园吗？

Mom：You don't have to. You must lie down and have a good rest. I will put a cool towel on your forehead to cool you down.

妈妈：不去了，你需要躺下好好休息。我先用凉毛巾敷在你的额头帮你降温。

Philip：OK, thanks, Mom!

飞飞：好的，谢谢妈妈!

词汇

headache ['hedeɪk] n. 头疼

medicine ['medɪsn] n. 药物

forehead ['fɔːhed] n. 额头

HAVE A COUGH

对话

Mom：Honey, you are not feeling well, aren't you?

妈妈：宝贝，你不舒服是吗？

Philip：I have been coughing since this morning.

飞飞：我从早上就一直咳嗽。

Mom：Do you have a sore throat?

妈妈：你嗓子疼吗？

Philip：Yes.

飞飞：是的。

Mom：Come here and take a temperature. It's not a fever.

妈妈：过来量一下体温。没有发烧。

Philip：Should I lie in bed?

飞飞：那我要躺在床上吗？

Mom：Well, lie down and have a rest. I'll bring you some water.

妈妈：嗯，躺下休息，我给你倒些水喝。

Philip：Can I still go outside and play today?

飞飞：我今天能出去玩吗？

Mom：It's very cold today. You'd better stay at home.

妈妈：今天外面很冷，你最好还是留在家里。

Philip：OK，Mom.

飞飞：好的，妈妈。

词汇

cough ［kɒf］ n. &v. 咳嗽

throat ［θrəʊt］ n. 喉咙

sore ［sɔː(r)］ adj. 疼痛的

GET RASHES

对话

Susan：What's the matter?

素琴：怎么了？

Mom：Phil has some red rashes on his body.

妈妈：飞飞身上有一些红疹子。

Susan：Did he take any medicine today?

素琴：他今天吃过什么药吗？

Mom：No，he didn't.

妈妈：没有吃药。

Susan：Is he allergic to any food?

素琴：他对什么食物过敏么？

Mom：He is allergic to peaches.

妈妈：他对桃子过敏。

Susan：Philip, what did you eat today in kindergarten?

素琴：飞飞，你今天在幼儿园都吃了什么东西啊？

Philip：I had rice, tomatoes, eggs and a peach.

飞飞：吃的米饭、西红柿、鸡蛋和一个桃子。

Mom：You got a lot of red rashes the last time you ate peaches. You must stay away from peaches.

妈妈：你上次吃桃子就起了很多红色的疹子，你得离桃子远点。

Susan：Don't worry. I'll keep an eye on him. If he is not feeling well, we take him to see a doctor.

素琴：别担心。我会盯着他。如果他感到不舒服，我们就带他去看医生。

词汇

rash ［ræʃ］ n. 疹子

allergic ［əˈlɜːdʒɪk］ adj. 过敏的

HAVE DIARRHEA

对话

Philip：Mom, I have a runny tummy.
飞飞：妈妈，我拉肚子了！

Mom：Philip, come here and sit down. When did it start? Is your tummy still sore?
妈妈：飞飞，过来坐下。你从什么时候开始拉肚子的？现在肚子还疼吗？

Philip：I'm not sure. I have already pooped several times. It's not sore now.
飞飞：我不确定。我已经拉了好几次了。现在肚子不疼。

Mom：Was your tummy sore before you went to the washroom?
妈妈：你去洗手间之前肚子疼吗？

Philip：Yes, Mom.
飞飞：是的，妈妈。

Mom：Any vomiting?
妈妈：吐过吗？

Philip：I'm not vomiting, but I'm sick at times.
飞飞：没吐过，但是有时我觉得恶心。

Mom：No worries. I will take you to see a doctor!
妈妈：别担心，我带你去看医生吧！

Philip：Mom, I don't want to take medicine!
飞飞：妈妈，我不想吃药！

Mom：You'll be fine if you take some medicine, and you can go to kindergarten and play with your friends!
妈妈：吃些药就会好了，你就能去幼儿园和小朋友一起玩了！

Philip：OK, Mom.
飞飞：好吧，妈妈。

词汇

washroom［ˈwɒʃruːm］n. 洗手间
vomit［ˈvɒmɪt］v. 呕吐

HAVE ECZEMA

对话

Philip：Susan, I'm terribly itchy!
飞飞：阿姨，我身上好痒啊！

Susan：You have a lot of red rashes on your neck and back.
素琴：你的脖子和后背起了好多小红疹子。

Philip：Scratch for me, Susan!
飞飞：帮我挠挠吧，阿姨！

Susan：No, sweetie. If your skin is scratched, it will hurt.
素琴：不行，宝贝。如果皮肤被抓破了，会疼的。

Philip：What can I do? It's terrible!
飞飞：怎么办啊？好难受啊！

Susan：I will help you take a shower and then put some ointment on your skin.
素琴：我帮你洗个澡，然后涂点药膏。

Philip：OK!
飞飞：好的！

词汇

eczema ［ˈeksɪmə］ n. 湿疹
terrible ［ˈterəbl］ adj. 令人极不快的
shower ［ˈʃaʊə(r)］ n. 淋浴
scratch ［skrætʃ］ v. 抓破；挠

HAVE CONSTIPATION

对话

Susan：Phil, Have you pooped this morning?
素琴：飞飞，你今天早上拉过便便了吗?

Philip：No.
飞飞：没有。

Susan：You didn't poop either yesterday.
素琴：你昨天也没有拉便便。

Philip：No, I didn't.
飞飞：是的，我没拉。

Susan：Do you want to poop now?
素琴：你现在想拉便便吗?

Philip：I don't want to poop.
飞飞：不想。

Susan：Do you feel bloated in your belly?
素琴：你觉得肚子胀吗?

Philip：I feel a little uncomfortable in my belly.
飞飞：我觉得肚子有一点不舒服。

Susan：You didn't drink much water in kindergarten, did you?
素琴：你在幼儿园没喝多少水，是吗?

Philip：I didn't drink any water in the afternoon.
飞飞：我下午都没喝水。

Susan：Phil, you should drink more water and eat more fruits, or you will not be able to poo!
素琴：飞飞，你要多喝水，多吃些水果，不然拉不出便便的。

Philip：OK, Susan, I've got it! I am going to grab some fruits. I will drink more water and eat more fruits.
飞飞：好的，阿姨，我知道了! 我现在就去拿些水果，以后多喝水，多吃水果。

Susan：Good kid!
素琴：好孩子!

词汇

bloated ［ˈbləʊtɪd］ adj. 胃胀的
grab ［græb］ vt. 拿，取

GET TOOTHACHE

对话

Mom：Are you OK? You don't look very well.
妈妈：你还好吗? 你看上去脸色不太好。

Philip：I have a toothache.
飞飞：我牙疼。

Mom：Oh my gosh! Do you have cavities? Open your mouth. Let me have a look!
妈妈：天啊! 你是不是长蛀牙了? 张

开嘴巴，妈妈看一下。

Philip：Ah—
飞飞：啊——

Mom：Phil, I see a hole in one of the teeth. We'd better see a dentist!
妈妈：飞飞，我看到一颗牙齿上有一个洞，我们去看医生吧！

Philip：No, I don't want to go. I don't have any problems with my teeth! I brush my teeth every day.
飞飞：不，我不去，我的牙齿没问题。我每天都刷牙的。

Mom：But you have a bad toothache.
妈妈：可你的牙齿很痛啊。

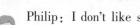
Philip：I don't like seeing dentists very much!
飞飞：我不太喜欢牙医！

Mom：Let's have a dental check-up first. If you have cavities, you should have timely treatment.
妈妈：咱们先检查一下牙齿，如果有蛀牙，要及时治疗。

Philip：But I'm scared.
飞飞：可是我害怕。

Mom：If you don't go to the dentist, your teeth will always be sore and you won't be able to eat delicious cookies any longer!
妈妈：如果你不去看牙医，你的牙齿会一直痛，这样就再也不能吃美味的饼干了！

Philip：No!
飞飞：不要！

Mom：Then Let's go to the dentist.
妈妈：那我们去看牙医吧。

Philip：OK.
飞飞：好吧。

词汇

toothache［ˈtuːθeɪk］n. 牙疼
dentist［ˈdentɪst］n. 牙医

CATCH A COLD

对话

Philip：Mom, I have a runny nose. Can you wipe it?
飞飞：妈妈。我流鼻涕了，帮我擦擦好吗？

Mom：When did you have a runny nose, sweetie?
妈妈：宝贝你什么时候开始流鼻涕的？

Philip：I had a runny nose in kindergarten today. My teacher helped me wipe my nose. Atishoo!
飞飞：今天在幼儿园就有，老师还帮我擦鼻涕了。阿嚏！

Mom：The temperature has dropped recently and you may have caught a cold. Have you had a headache and a sore throat?
妈妈：最近气温下降，你可能感冒了。头疼吗？嗓子疼吗？

Philip：No, only runny nose.
飞飞：没有，只是流鼻涕。

Mom：You should drink more water, and eat more vegetables and fruits, which will help you get rid of those small bacteria!

妈妈：飞飞，你要多喝水，多吃蔬菜、水果，这样能帮你赶走小细菌哦！

Philip：I'd like to drink some juice.

飞飞：我想喝果汁。

Mom：OK. Is orange juice OK?

妈妈：好。橙汁可以吗？

Philip：Good!

飞飞：太好了！

词汇

wipe［waɪp］v. 擦拭

bacteria［bækˈtɪərɪə］n. 细菌

HAVE A NOSE BLEED

对话

Susan：What's wrong, Philip? Is your nose bleeding?

素琴：飞飞，你怎么了？鼻子流血了？

Philip：When a boy was playing football, the ball hit me on the nose.

飞飞：有个小男孩踢球，把球踢到我鼻子上了。

Susan：Come and sit down. I will pinch the lower part of your nose.

素琴：过来坐下，我会轻轻捏住你鼻子的下面。

Philip：OK.

飞飞：好的。

Susan：Lean forward to avoid swallowing the blood and breathe through your mouth.

素琴：身体前倾，这样就不会把血吞下去，用嘴呼吸。

Philip：How long does it take?

飞飞：需要多长时间？

Susan：A full 10 minutes.

素琴：整10分钟。

Philip：Does it work?

飞飞：有用吗？

Susan：We have to wait and see. It may help to apply ice across the bridge of your nose. Pinch your nose, and I'll get some ice.

素琴：我们需要等着看。用冰敷在你的鼻梁上会有作用，捏住你的鼻子，我去拿一些冰。

Philip：Sure.

飞飞：好。

词汇

bleed［bliːd］vi. 出血

lean［liːn］vi. 倾斜

SCALD YOURSELF

对话

Philip：Susan, come here! It hurts!

飞飞：素琴，快过来，好疼啊！

Susan：What's wrong, Philip?

素琴：怎么了？飞飞？

Philip：I burnt my hands with hot water! Ouch!

飞飞：热水烫手了，疼！

Susan：No worries. Go to the bathroom with me. Let's flush your hands with cool water now.

素琴：别怕。我带你去卫生间，用凉水冲一下手。

Philip：Susan, I'm scared.

飞飞：素琴，我怕。

Susan：It will be fine. Cool running water will stop the burning process and cool the burn.

素琴：会没事的，流动的凉水可以防止烫伤发展，为烫伤部位降温。

Philip：How long does it take?

飞飞：需要多长时间？

Susan：20 minutes.

素琴：20 分钟。

词汇

scald [skɔːld] v. （沸水等）烫伤

burn [bɜːn] v. 烫伤；n. 烫伤

HAVE INDIGESTION

对话

Philip：Susan, I'm not feeling well.

飞飞：素琴，我不舒服。

Susan：What did you eat in the kindergarten today?

素琴：你在幼儿园吃的什么晚餐？

Philip：I ate ten stuffed bun and a bowl of soup.

飞飞：我吃了十个包子喝了一碗汤。

Susan：You ate a lot of food. It seems like indigestion.

素琴：你吃了好多食物，似乎是消化不良了。

Philip：What should I do?

飞飞：我该怎么办？

Susan：You'll need to take some medicine. It can help you with digestion, or you will still feel unwell.

素琴：你最好吃点药。可以帮助你消化，要不然会一直不舒服。

Philip：Is it bitter?

飞飞：药苦吗？

Susan：Actually, it's not bitter. It's sweet.

素琴：这个药不苦的，是甜的。

Philip：Well, I'll take it.

飞飞：那好吧，我吃。

词汇

digestion [daɪˈdʒestʃən] n. 消化

actually [ˈæktʃuəli] adv. 实际上

discomfort [dɪsˈkʌmfət] n. 不适

HAVE ANAEMIA

对话

Mom：Hello, doctor! I took my daughter for a health examination this morning. Here is the results of her blood tests.

妈妈：医生您好！我今天上午带女儿做了体检。这是她的验血结果。

Doctor：Her hemoglobin level is slightly lower than normal. It is 105 g/L.

医生：血红蛋白是 105g/L，略低于正常水平。

Mom：Is it necessary for her to take medicine？

妈妈：她需要吃药吗？

Doctor：Don't worry. It's not serious. She doesn't have to take any medicine. My advice is to eat more iron-rich food to improve her nutrition.

医生：别担心，不是特别严重。暂时不用吃药。我的建议是多吃含铁丰富的食物来改善她的营养。

Mom：Such as？

妈妈：比如？

Doctor：Animal livers, spinach, red meat and so on. Encourage her to eat more fresh vegetables and fruits, as well as high-protein food. Repeat CBC test three months later.

医生：动物肝脏、菠菜、红肉等。平时多给她吃新鲜的蔬菜、水果和高蛋白食物。三个月之后复查血常规。

Mom：Thanks, doctor.

妈妈：谢谢医生。

词汇

anaemia ［əˈniːmɪə］ n. 贫血
hemoglobin ［ˌhiːməˈɡləʊbɪn］ n. 血红蛋白
nutrition ［njuˈtrɪʃn］ n. 营养
encourage ［ɪnˈkʌrɪdʒ］ v. 鼓励
CBC 全血细胞计数（血常规）

HAVE A HEADACHE

对话

Philip：Mom, I'm not feeling well!

飞飞：妈妈，我难受！

Mom：What's the matter, honey？

妈妈：怎么了，宝贝？

Philip：I have a headache.

飞飞：我觉得头疼。

Mom：Honey, you went to bed at 11:30 p. m. Headaches can be caused by a lack of sleep.

妈妈：宝贝，你晚上 11 点半才睡。头痛可能是睡眠不足引起的。

Philip：Do I need to take medicine？

飞飞：我需要吃药吗？

Mom：First, let's try some home remedies. If your headaches are not relieved, I'll take you to a hospital.

妈妈：我们先尝试一些家庭疗法，如果你的头痛没有缓解，我就带你去医院。

Philip：What are the home remedies？

飞飞：家庭疗法是什么呀？

Mom：Use a cold compress. A cold compress may help soothe your pain. And healthy snacks may help to reduce headache symptoms.

妈妈：使用冷敷法。冷敷可能有助于缓解疼痛。健康的零食也有助于减轻头痛症状。

Philip: I'd like some cherries.
飞飞：我想吃樱桃。

Mom: OK.
妈妈：好的。

词汇

compress ['kɒmpres] n. 敷布
remedy ['remədi] n. 疗法

GET ORAL ULCER

对话

Ann: Susan, my mouth hurts.
安安：素琴，我的嘴巴好痛。

Susan: Oh, my dear, can you open your mouth for me?
素琴：哦，宝贝，你能张嘴让我看看吗？

Ann: Ah—
安安：啊——

Susan: Can I have a look at your lips sweetheart? You have an oral ulcer.
素琴：宝贝，我能看一下你的嘴唇吗？你的嘴里有口腔溃疡了。

Ann: What is an oral ulcer?
安安：什么口腔溃疡？

Susan: That means there is a small wound in your mouth.
素琴：就是你的嘴巴里破了一块。

Ann: What can I do with it?
安安：那要怎么办啊？

Susan: You need to take more fruits and vegetables. It will heal soon.
素琴：你要多吃水果和蔬菜。很快就能好了。

Ann: I want apples.
安安：我要吃苹果。

Susan: OK, sweetheart. I am going to wash apples for you.
素琴：好的宝贝，我去给你洗苹果。

Ann: Thank you, Susan.
安安：谢谢你，素琴。

词汇

oral ['ɔːrəl] adj. 口腔的
ulcer ['ʌlsə(r)] n. 溃疡
lip [lɪp] n. 嘴唇

GET HYPOGLYCEMIA

对话

Susan: What is wrong? You look pale.
素琴：您怎么了？您的脸色很苍白。

Grandma: I don't know. I am feeling a little dizzy.
姥姥：我也不知道，我觉得有些头晕。

Susan: Here, take a seat. Did you take the insulin shot this afternoon?
素琴：您快坐下。您中午有没有注射胰岛素？

Grandma: Yes, I did. I took 8 units as my doctor told me.
姥姥：有啊。我按照医生告诉我的注射了8个单位的胰岛素。

94

Susan：Did you have anything for lunch?

素琴：那您有没有吃饭呢?

 Grandma：Not yet. I just had a cookie.

姥姥：还没有。我只吃了一块饼干。

 Susan：You must to take a blood sugar test right now. You might have hypoglycemia.

素琴：你得赶快测个血糖。你可能是低血糖了。

 Grandma：Am I? Could you please take a test for me?

姥姥：是吗? 你能帮我测一下吗?

 Susan：Oh, your blood sugar level is only 4. That's quite low for you. Please wait for me. I will bring you a glass of orange juice.

素琴：哦,你的血糖只有4,那对你来说确实太低了。请等一下,我去给你倒一杯橙汁。

 Grandma：Well. Thank you, Susan.

姥姥：好的,谢谢你素琴!

 Susan：Have some juice. I'll be by your side until you blood sugar level returns to normal.

素琴：喝橙汁吧。我会陪在你身边,直到你的血糖水平恢复正常。

 Grandma：I'm grateful to have you here.

姥姥：你能在这我很感激。

 Susan：You should be fine now. Please remember to have meals after taking insulin shots. Otherwise, it's easy for you to get hypoglycemia.

 素琴：你现在应该没事了。以后你打完胰岛素要及时吃饭啊,不然很容易发生低血糖的。

 Grandma：I will, Susan. Thanks a lot.

姥姥：我会的,素琴。太感谢了。

词汇

hypoglycemia［ˌhaɪpəʊɡlaɪˈsiːmiə］n. 低血糖

pale［peɪl］adj. 苍白的

dizzy［ˈdɪzi］adj. 眩晕的

insulin［ˈɪnsjəlɪn］n. 胰岛素

unit［ˈjuːnɪt］n. 单位

CATCH PNEUMONIA

对话

 Susan：Hi, Tracy. It's been a long time since we last met.

素琴：嗨,崔蕾,好久不见。

 Tracy：Hey, Susan. Haven't seen you for a long time. Why are you here in the hospital?

崔蕾：嗨,素琴,好久没见过你了,你为什么来医院了?

 Susan：I have come here to see Ann. She's ill.

素琴：我是来看望安安的。她生病了。

 Tracy：Ann is a lovely child.

崔蕾：安安是个可爱的孩子。

 Susan：She caught pneumonia. She has been coughing for a week, and she was taken to this hospital yesterday because she had a high fever.

素琴：她得了肺炎已经咳嗽一周了。因为昨天发高烧，她被送来医院。

Tracy：Oh, poor child. How is she doing right now?

崔蕾：哦，可怜的孩子。她现在怎么样了？

Susan：She's been put on antibiotics. Now she has no fever, and she is more energetic.

素琴：她已经服用了抗生素。现在已经不再发烧了，人也精神了许多。

Tracy：I hope she will get better soon.

崔蕾：希望她快点好起来。

Susan：Yeah, when she was full of energy, she was the cutest.

素琴：是啊，她活力满满的时候是最可爱的。

词汇

pneumonia [njuːˈməʊnɪə] n. 肺炎

antibiotic [ˌæntɪbaɪˈɒtɪk] n. 抗生素

energy [ˈenədʒi] n. 精力，活力

PILLOW BALDNESS

对话

Grandma：Ann, my cute girl, are you at home?

姥姥：安安，我的小可爱，你在家吗？

Ann：I'm here, grandma.

安安：我在这呢，姥姥。

Grandma：My little cutie is even prettier, with black waterfalls hair.

姥姥：我的小可爱更漂亮了，满头瀑布一样的黑发。

Mom：Her hair is getting thicker and thicker, and I can't tell how thin it used to be.

妈妈：她的头发越来越浓密了，我都想不起来以前有多稀少了。

Grandma：It's normal for children to have thin hair when they are young. As long as there is no pillow baldness.

姥姥：孩子小时候头发不多也正常，只要没有枕秃就行。

Mom：Have I ever had pillow baldness?

妈妈：我曾经得过枕秃吗？

Grandma：Yes, as a baby, you used to rub your head against the pillow, resulting in pillow baldness.

姥姥：是啊，你小时候经常把头在枕头上蹭来蹭去，导致枕秃。

Ann：What happened later?

安安：后来怎样了？

Grandma：Her hair loss stopped after taking the vitamin D supplement.

姥姥：在服用了维生素 D 补充剂后她就停止了脱发。

词汇

pillow [ˈpɪləʊ] n. 枕头

bald [bɔːld] adj. 秃顶的

rub [rʌb] v. 摩擦

vitamin [ˈvɪtəmɪn] n. 维生素

CATCH HERPETIC PHARYNGITIS

对话

Philip：Susan, I'm sick.
飞飞：素琴，我想吐。

Susan：Phil, what's wrong?
素琴：飞飞，你怎么了？

Philip：I have a headache and I feel very cold.
飞飞：我头痛，而且很冷。

Susan：Honey, can I take your temperature?
素琴：宝贝，我帮你测一个体温好吗？

Philip：Alright Susan.
飞飞：好的素琴。

Susan：Honey, your temperature is high. You have a fever.
素琴：宝贝，你的体温很高，你发烧了。

Philip：Susan, my throat is sore.
飞飞：素琴，我的喉咙疼。

Susan：Honey, I think you need to see a doctor.
素琴：宝贝，我觉得你需要去看医生。

Doctor：What's the problem?
医生：怎么了？

Susan：Philip vomited four times at home today. His temperature was 39.2℃. He also had a headache and a sore throat.

素琴：今天飞飞在家吐了 4 次。体温 39.2 摄氏度，他的头和嗓子都疼。

Doctor：Has he had any food today?
医生：他今天有吃过什么东西吗？

Susan：No, he had a bad appetite and only drank a little milk at noon today.
素琴：没有，他今天食欲非常差，只在中午喝了一点牛奶。

Doctor：Are there any other symptoms?
医生：还有其他症状吗？

Mom：I have seen his throat. It looks red.
妈妈：我看他的嗓子很红。

Doctor：OK. Let's take a look at little Phil. Phil, can you show me your throat?
医生：好的，让我们来看看小飞飞。飞飞，能让我看看你的嗓子吗？

Philip：Ah——
飞飞：啊——

Doctor：His throat is red and swollen, and there is a vesicular rash on the back of his pharynx.
医生：他的嗓子红肿，咽后部有水疱疹。

Mom：What disease does he get?
妈妈：他得了什么病？

Doctor：He gets herpetic pharyngitis.
医生：疱疹性咽峡炎。

词汇

herpetic pharyngitis 疱疹性咽峡炎
appetite [ˈæpɪtaɪt] n. 食欲
symptom [ˈsɪmptəm] n. 症状
swollen [ˈswəʊlən] adj. 肿胀的

vesicula rash   水泡疹

DEAL WITH WOUNDS

对话

Susan：What's going on, Philip?
素琴：怎么了，飞飞？

Philip：Susan, my hand hurts.
飞飞：素琴，我的手好痛。

Susan：Oh, Phil, your hand is bleeding.
素琴：哦，飞飞，你的手在流血。

Philip：Susan, it hurts!
飞飞：素琴，好痛啊！

Susan：You must have scratched your hand when you played with scissors. I'm going to stop bleeding.
素琴：一定是你刚刚玩剪刀的时候划伤了手。我先帮你止血。

Philip：Please help me.
飞飞：快帮帮我吧。

Susan：I'm going to get the first aid kit. Do not move please.
素琴：我去拿急救包。不要动哦。

Susan：First, we need to clean the cut. I'll wash your hand with soap and water.
素琴：我们先要清洁伤口。我要用肥皂给你洗手。

Philip：Ouch. It hurts.
飞飞：好痛。

Susan：To stop the bleeding, I'll press the bandage on your hand.
素琴：我要把绷带按在你手上止血。

Philip：The bleeding is stopped.
飞飞：血止住了。

Susan：Next, spread a small amount of antibacterial ointment across the cut to prevent an infection. Then cover it with a Band-Aid.
素琴：接下来，在伤口上涂少量的抗菌药膏，以防止感染。然后用创可贴盖住。

Philip：Thank you Susan.
飞飞：谢谢你，素琴。

词汇

aid［eɪd］n. 帮助
kit［kɪt］n. 工具箱
wound［wuːnd］n. 伤口
Band – Aid 邦迪创可贴

FALL OFF THE BED

对话

Ann：Daddy, Phil fell off the bed.
安安：爸爸，飞飞从床上掉下来了。

Dad：Phil, are you alright?
爸爸：飞飞，你没事吧？

Philip：Dad, my right hand hurts.
飞飞：爸爸，我的右手好痛。

Dad：Honey, don't be afraid. Can you turn your right hand around slowly? Is it possible to move it?
爸爸：宝贝，别怕，你能慢慢转过右手来吗？能动吗？

Philip：Dad, my hands can move, but it hurts.

飞飞：爸爸，我的手能动，但是很痛。

Dad：Honey，can I take a look at your right hand?

爸爸：宝贝，能让爸爸看看你的右手吗？

Philip：Ouch！

飞飞：好痛！

Dad：Let's go to hospital.

爸爸：我们去医院吧。

Philip：I really don't like hospitals.

飞飞：我真不喜欢去医院。

词汇

turn around （使）调转方向

HAVE A CHEST PAIN

对话

Grandpa：Susan！Susan！

姥爷：素琴！素琴！

Susan：What is wrong? It appears that you are in pain.

素琴：您怎么了？您看起来很痛苦。

Grandpa：My chest and left shoulder are both in pain.

姥爷：我胸和左肩都很痛。

（Grandpa suddenly appears pale, his hands covering his chest and a lot of cold sweat streaming down his brow.）

（姥爷突然面色苍白，手捂胸口，额头冒出大量冷汗）

Susan：Are you alright? Take a deep breath.

素琴：您还好吗？深呼吸。

（Grandpa does not answer, his facial expression is very painful）

（姥爷并没有回答，表情非常痛苦）

Susan：Do you have nitroglycerin in your bag?

素琴：您包里有没有硝酸甘油？

（Grandpa shakes his head）

（姥爷摇摇头）

Susan：God！Lie down on the sofa，please. I'm going to call 120.

素琴：天啊！躺在沙发上。我去打120。

（Susan picks up the phone on the table next to her and dials）

（素琴拿起旁边桌子上的手机，拨号）

Susan：Hello，an elderly man had unbearable chest pain，probably a heart attack. Please send an ambulance to help us.

素琴：你好，有一名老人出现了难以忍受的胸痛，没有外伤，可能是心脏病发作。请派救护车来帮助我们。

120：Help is on the way and will arrive at your place soon. Please let the elderly rest on the ground and do not let him move.

120：救护车已经派出，很快会到您家里，请让老人平卧休息，减少活动。

词汇

chest [tʃest] n. 胸部

shoulder [ˈʃəʊldə(r)] n. 肩

sweat [swet] n. 汗水

brow [braʊ] n. 额头

nitroglycerin [ˌnaɪtrəʊˈɡlɪsəriːn] n. 硝酸甘油

99

unbearable［ʌnˈbeərəbl］adj. 难以忍受的

heart attack　心脏病发作

ambulance［ˈæmbjələns］n. 救护车

HAVE A STOMACHACHE

对话

Ann：Susan, I've got a sore tummy.
安安：素琴，我的肚子好痛。

Susan：What's wrong, sweetheart? Where is the pain?
素琴：怎么了宝贝，哪里痛？

Ann：Here.
安安：这里。

Susan：Sweetheart, did you just eat a lot of ice cream?
素琴：宝贝，你刚刚是不是吃了很多冰激凌？

Ann：Not a lot. I had only half of the cup.
安安：没有很多。我只吃了半盒。

Susan：Sweetheart, that's a large cup of ice cream. You've eaten too much.
素琴：宝贝，那可是很大一盒冰激凌啊，你吃得太多了。

Ann：Susan, what should I do?
安安：素琴，我怎么办呀？

Susan：I will get a hot-water bag to see if it will help.
素琴：我去拿个热水袋，看看会不会好一点。

Ann：Alright.
安安：好吧。

Susan：Sweetheart, are you feeling better?
素琴：宝贝，你好一点了吗？

Ann：The pain is gone.
安安：不痛了。

Susan：Sweetheart, don't eat too much ice cream at a time.
素琴：宝贝，不能一次吃那么多冰激凌了哦。

Ann：I will not. I swear.
安安：我发誓再也不会了。

词汇

swear［sweə(r)］vt. 发誓

DON'T CHOKE

对话

Philip：Mom, I want to eat jelly.
飞飞：妈妈，我想吃果冻了。

Mom：Honey, jelly is an unhealthy food, and it's very dangerous. Would you rather have something else?
妈妈：宝贝，果冻是不健康的食物，而且很危险，你愿意吃点别的东西吗？

Philip：Why, Many children eat jelly.
飞飞：为什么？很多小朋友都会吃果冻的啊。

Mom：Because jelly is very slippery. If it's not well chewed, it's easy to slide into the windpipe. Then you can't breathe. So it's dangerous.
妈妈：因为果冻很滑，如果嚼得不好就容易滑到气管里。你就没有办法喘气了，所以很危险。

Philip：But I can chew it well.
飞飞：那我可以好好嚼啊。

Mom：Still, I'm worried. Jason had been in the hospital for a long time because he was choked by jelly.
妈妈：我还是很担心。之前杰森就曾经因为吃果冻窒息进了医院，住了很久。

Philip：Oh, I don't want to be in the hospital. Mom, can I have strawberries?
飞飞：哦，我可不想住院。妈妈，那我可以吃草莓吗？

Mom：Of course, honey. You should also chew strawberries well when you eat them.
妈妈：当然了宝贝。吃草莓的时候也要嚼碎哦。

Philip：OK.
飞飞：好的。

词汇

jelly ['dʒeli] n. 果冻
chew [tʃuː] v. 咀嚼
windpipe ['wɪndpaɪp] n. 气管
choke [tʃəʊk] v. （使）窒息

练 习

CHAPTER ONE　HAVE A MEAL

一、根据课文内容填空

1. Because you need water to _____ your body.

2. This apple looks very _____!

3. You need to drink more water, eat _____ food and hot soup.

二、用所给单词的正确形式填空

1. Don't forget to _____（wash）the apple before you eat it!

2. How about _____（watch）TV after dinner?

3. Some food cannot be _____（keep）in the fridge, such as bananas and mangoes.

三、选择

1. You may _____ some water.
   A. drink　　　　B. drinks
   C. drinking　　 D. drank

2. Is there anything to eat when Ann _____ back at night?
   A. come　　　　B. comes
   C. came　　　　D. coming

四、翻译句子

1. 你口渴吗?

2. 这是什么水果?

3. 这可真是个好主意!

4. 哇，好丰盛的饭菜!

5. 饭前要洗手哦。

CHAPTER TWO　DAILY ACTIVITIES

一、根据课文内容填空

1. Phil, let's put on our raincoats and boots, and get _____, OK?

2. We need to go to the community hospital for a routine physical _____.

3. Watch out for the _____ floor, children.

二、用所给单词的正确形式填空

1. _____（Wait）in line to order food is a virtue, so we should wait.

2. You've _____（learn）how to cross the street properly and safely.

3. The Super Flying is a mailman who _____（help）to make dreams come true.

三、选择

1. Let me help you hang _____ the clothes.
   A. over　　　　B. around
   C. up　　　　　D. down

2. Wow, Ann, you're really good _____

drawing.

A. at   B. in

C. for   D. with

四、翻译句子

1. 妈妈，我想去堆雪人。

2. 安安，今天你得去打疫苗了。

3. 能讲个故事给我听吗？

4. 妈妈，你今晚能跟我一起睡吗？

5. 这是宝宝的眼睛、耳朵和嘴。

CHAPTER THREE INDOOR GAMES

一、根据课文内容填空

1. Could you do me a _____, please?

2. Oh, there is a _____ little boy.

3. Since it fell down, let's _____ the blocks.

二、用所给单词的正确形式填空

1. _____ (keep) him safe as he slides down.

2. Let's _____ (switch) roles.

3. I can't wait to _____ (paint) it.

三、选择

1. When you see the red light, you have to _____.

    A. go   B. stop

    C. cross the road   D. wait

2. Do you want to _____?

    A. give it a shot   B. give it

    C. shot it   D. give it shot

四、翻译句子

1. 让我们随着音乐摇摆。

2. 真是一个好主意！

3. 我擅长跳跃。

4. 祝贺你目标达成。

5. 好酷的纸飞机！

CHAPTER FOUR OUTDOOR ACTIVITIES

一、根据课文内容填空

1. I'd like to _____ my bike.

2. You are a very _____ seller.

3. We are going to pick strawberries in the _____ today.

二、用所给单词的正确形式填空

1. Because we are going to _____ (have) picnic there.

2. That is to sell something we don't use anymore in our family and _____ (donate) the money to those who need it.

3. _____ (insert) the tips of each pole into these eyelets.

三、选择

1. I've decided to sell this toy rabbit _____ I have a similar one.

    A. unless   B. so

    C. because   D. because of

2. Daddy is _____ duty today.

    A. in   B. at

    C. of   D. on

四、翻译句子

1. 你想要一些帮助吗？

2. 我要享受一下这温暖的阳光。

3. 每个初学者都是从跌倒中学习的。

4. 我们今天要去果园采摘草莓。

5. 这是我见过的最棒的雪人！

CHAPTER FIVE   HEALTH CARE

一、根据课文内容填空

1. Daddy, Phil _____ the bed.

2. I will put a _____ on your forehead to help you cool down.

3. My _____ and left shoulder are both in pain.

二、用所给单词的正确形式填空

1. I am not _____ (feel) very well!

2. Any _____ (vomit)?

3. If the skin is _____ (scratch), it hurts.

三、选择

1. If you don't go to the dentist, your teeth will always be sore and you won't _____ eat delicious cookies any longer!

    A. can   B. able

    C. be able   D. be able to

2. Since _____ have you had a runny nose, sweetie?

    A. when   B. where

    C. how   D. what

四、翻译句子

1. 妈妈，我不想吃药！

2. 你嗓子疼吗？

3. 我真不喜欢去医院。

4. 我发誓再也不会了。

5. 吃草莓的时候也要嚼碎哦。